The Dental Foundation Interview Guide
with Situational Judgement Tests

The Dental Foundation Interview Guide

with Situational Judgement Tests

Zahid Siddique

Shivana Anand

Helena Lewis-Greene

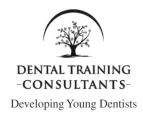

DENTAL TRAINING
-CONSULTANTS-

Developing Young Dentists

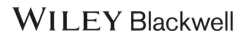

WILEY Blackwell

Library of Congress Cataloging-in-Publication Data

Names: Siddique, Zahid, 1985- , author. | Anand, Shivana, 1990- , author. |
  Lewis-Greene, Helena, 1954- , author.
Title: Situational judgment tests for dentists : the DF1 guidebook / Dr.
  Zahid Siddique, Dr. Shivana Anand, Dr. Helena Lewis-Greene.
Description: Chichester, West Sussex ; Hoboken, NJ : John Wiley & Sons Inc.,
  2016. | Includes bibliographical references and index.
Identifiers: LCCN 2015043956 | ISBN 9781119109143 (pbk.)
Subjects: | MESH: Education, Dental, Graduate–Great Britain. |
  Dentists–psychology–Great Britain. | Educational Measurement–Great
  Britain. | Employment–Great Britain. | Judgment–Great Britain.
Classification: LCC RK76 | NLM WU 20 | DDC 617.60071/141–dc23 LC record available at
  http://lccn.loc.gov/2015043956

A catalogue record for this book is available from the British Library.

Wiley also publishes its books in a variety of electronic formats. Some content that appears in print may
not be available in electronic books.

Cover image: © Getty/Westend61

Set in 9/12pt, MeridienLTStd by SPi Global, Chennai, India.
Printed and bound in Malaysia by Vivar Printing Sdn Bhd

1 2017

Contents

Preface

There are several books available on medical situational judgement tests (SJTs) but none for dentistry. Situational judgement test questions were introduced as part of the DFT application interview process in 2013. A relatively new concept in dentistry, SJTs have been widely used in industry as part of the selection criteria for professionals. We wanted to provide students with a selection of subject-specific SJT questions to help with their DFT preparations. Guidance for preparation has been put together by recently qualified dentists who understand the pressures that undergraduate study can impose. We hope that this book will be useful in helping all students gain experience with SJTs, leadership and management as well as clinical scenarios.

The DFT application process is highly competitive. Simply put, the higher the ranking the better the chance of getting your first choice placement. We hope that this book gives you all the information that you need in order to achieve this goal.

The SJTs in this book were verified and standardized by a group of dentists and are answered in accordance to their opinion and expertise.

Acknowledgements

Thank you to Mr Raj Rattan for his continued support and mentorship throughout this process. Thank you to Professor Dunne our Professor in Primary Dental Care at King's College London Dental Institute for his support and guidance from the beginning.

A huge thank you to some of the panel members who include:

Dr Razaullah Ahmed BDS
Dr Keshvi Patel BDS MJDF RCS(Lon)
Dr Nirupy Shanmugathas BDS MJDF RCS(Lon)
Dr Simrun Chowdhary BDS MJDF RCS(Lon)

CHAPTER 1

What is dental foundation training?

Dental foundation training is a year when dental graduates across the United Kingdom embark on a period of relevant employment general dental practitioners under a contract of service by approved educational supervisors to provide a wide range of dental care and treatment. The successful completion of the DF1 year is mandatory for those who want to work in the NHS as part of their future dental career. Dental foundation training (DF1) introduces new graduates to general practice and gives them a protected environment in which to work and enhance the basic dental skills achieved through their BDS degree under the supervision of a educational supervisor practitioner. The educational supervisor's role is to help and support the dental foundation trainee in all aspects of employment and provide continuous academic development through tutorials. The DF1 trainees also attend weekly study days outside of their general practice with the aim and objective of enhancing clinical and administrative competence and promoting high standards through relevant postgraduate training. The following competencies are included within the DFT curricula:

- to enable the dental practitioner to practise and improve dental practitioner's skills;
- to introduce the dental practitioner to all aspects of dental practice in primary care;
- to identify the dental practitioner's personal strengths and weaknesses and balance them through a planned programme of training;
- to promote oral health and the quality of dental care for patients;
- to develop and implement peer- and self-review and promote awareness of the need for professional education, training and audit as a continuing process;
- to demonstrate that the dental practitioner is working within the General Dental Council's (GDC's) standard guidelines.

Excerpts from the National Health Service (Performers Lists) (England) Regulations 2013, found at http://www.legislation.gov.uk/uksi/2013/335/pdfs/uksi_20130335_en.pdf (accessed 24 February 2016).

The Dental Foundation Interview Guide: with Situational Judgement Tests, First Edition.
Zahid Siddique, Shivana Anand and Helena Lewis-Greene.
© 2017 John Wiley & Sons, Ltd. Published 2017 by John Wiley & Sons, Ltd.

CHAPTER 2

The application process

DF1 recruitment process

All DF1 training vacancies are allocated through a centralized process for England, Northern Ireland and Wales. The online application process usually opens in the month of September for all UK-based **year 5 dental students** and EU graduates or overseas dentists.

The recruitment process is split in two stages:

- **First stage** – trainees are first allocated a particular DFT (dental foundation training) scheme. This is based on their DFT interview score ranking. The higher the candidates' ranking scores, the greater is the likelihood of them obtaining their first scheme preference and so forth.

- **Second stage** – trainees are allocated a particular practice in spring / summer of the following year. The individual practices are allocated through the DFT interview ranking scores, so those with the highest scores will receive their first preference practice and so forth. Some schemes carry out second-round interviews, where an algorithm is used to pair up trainee preferences with educational supervisor preferences.

The Dental Foundation Interview Guide: with Situational Judgement Tests, First Edition.
Zahid Siddique, Shivana Anand and Helena Lewis-Greene.
© 2017 John Wiley & Sons, Ltd. Published 2017 by John Wiley & Sons, Ltd.

Table 2.1 data collected for the application years 2011/12 and 2012/13 from COPDEND.

Numbers	2011/12 England and Wales	EEA	United Kingdom	ROW	2012/13 England and Wales	EEA	United Kingdom	ROW
Places Total	927				978			
Applicants Total	1190	101	1044	45	1172	110	1031	31
Applicants eligible and short listed	1145	97	1042	6	1153	109	1027	17
Applicants interviewed	1110	86	1018	6	1138	104	1021	13
Applicants offered place	940	47	889	4	1040	77	953	10
Applicants accepted offer	928	42	882	4	978	58	914	6
Applicants not accepted offer	12	5	7	0	18	13	3	2
Applicants not offered a place	48	13	35	0	55	11	41	3

Notes: *EEA – European Economic Area; ROW – Rest of the World

It is important to understand that the DFT application process is competitive. The number of DFT training places is generally linked to the number of final-year students but **places cannot be guaranteed for all UK graduates** and it is therefore of utmost importance that all students give themselves the best opportunity to secure a place.

Over the past few years the number of candidates applying has exceeded the number of DF1 positions available with EU and oversees dental applicants also applying.

Table 2.1 shows the data collected for the application years 2011/12 and 2012/13 from the Committee of Postgraduate Dental Deans and Directors (COPDEND).

How to apply

London application process

The London deanery and COPDEND change the application process on a yearly basis. It is always beneficial to look at the guidance notes released by COPDEND on the London deanery web site beforehand at http://www.lpmde.ac.uk/ (accessed 22 November 2015).

Scotland application process

See below.

Key dates

COPDEND has the right to change the recruitment process on a yearly basis. Table 2.2 is a proposed timeline for recruitment with guideline months.

Table 2.3 gives the selection centre interview venues across the United Kingdom.

DF1 schemes – where to work

A component of the DF1 application process involves choosing DF1 scheme area preferences around the United Kingdom. In 2014, applicants were asked to rank

Table 2.2 Proposed recruitment timetable.

Applications open	25 August 2015
Applications close	22 September 2015
Interview window	16 – 20 November 2015
Preferencing of schemes opens	8 December 2015
Preferencing of schemes closes	15 December 2015
Initial offers out by	06 January 2016
2nd round offers	06 July 2016
Placements commence	March 2016 and September 2016

Table 2.3 Selection centre interview venues.

Centre	Venue	Dental schools covered
London	London Recruitment Events Centre	King's College London Queen Mary University of London
Bristol	Bristol Marriott Hotel, City Centre	Bristol University Cardiff University Peninsula College of Dentistry
Manchester	Reebok Stadium, Bolton	University of Central Lancaster University of Liverpool University of Manchester
Birmingham	West Bromwich Albion	University of Birmingham University of Sheffield
Belfast	Ramada Hotel, Shaw's Bridge, Belfast	Queen's University, Belfast
Newcastle	Newcastle United Football Club	Newcastle University University of Leeds

their scheme preferences via the UK Offers System, which was done separately from the submission of their online application form for their original DF1 application. Candidates will be emailed with information regarding their interview date (which they must confirm within 48 hours) and full instructions on how to complete scheme preferences, including use of the UK offers system. This involves logging into the system approximately 3 weeks after the interview and submitting their scheme area preference. The submission for schemes is open for 7 days – after this period submissions cannot be made.

The London Deanery usually produces an information sheet about the available schemes for that year. It is of utmost importance that candidates take time to consider all the schemes and their locations. Due to the competitive nature of the application process it is imperative that the candidates give themselves the best possible opportunity to obtain a DF1 job offer. These opportunities can decrease if candidates limit the number of schemes they are willing to work in. If they do not rank one of the schemes they will automatically forfeit their place, even if a position is available. However, it should also be noted that there is no point in candidates ranking a scheme if they are absolutely certain that they are not willing to work in that region. The rationale for this is that if they do rank such a region and are offered a place within it, they will not be offered an alternative, or be given an opportunity to swap, if they decline the offer. We therefore advise candidates to try to be as flexible as possible when ranking schemes to give themselves the best opportunity to secure a DF1 job.

It is also important to note that, at this stage of the application process, candidates will only be given information regarding their scheme locations and not the locations of the actual training practices as they are not approved until spring / summer and can change on an annual basis. Some schemes cover a large geographical area and the distance between practices within a scheme can take over an hour to commute. The deanery will only provide detailed information about practices once they have all been approved; however, it might be possible to see the previous year's information regarding individual practices on its web site.

Once candidates have accepted their scheme in the beginning of January, they will have an option to 'upgrade' or 'accept' the offer. If they choose to accept, their deanery will be notified of their acceptance and their place for the DF1 year will be confirmed. If they choose to 'upgrade', then on the last day of January their scheme will either be upgraded to a higher choice or the candidate will stay in the same scheme.

Here are some useful points to consider when choosing where to work:

1 **Travelling to work**
    ◦ How far are you willing to travel to work?
    ◦ Do you drive? Will it be feasible to drive to work – Congestion charge? Parking?

- If you don't drive will you need to relocate close to a train / tube station? Will you need to relocate to make your commute to work easier?

2 **Finance**
  - How expensive will your living accommodation be in certain regions?
  - Will living at home be more suitable?
  - How expensive will your commute be?
  - Do you have any family commitments or are supporting any children? If so, consider childcare and school arrangements.

3 **Social life**
  - It is important that the location and environment you choose to work in provide a suitable social lifestyle outside of work, which caters for your individual needs.

4 **It is only for one year**
  - Always take into consideration all factors. However, this is your opportunity to shine, build your CV, gain extra experience and make mistakes from which you will learn.
  - Chose an environment in which you will feel comfortable to grow professionally and personally. Flexibility is key and it *is* only for one year.

5 **Location**
  - It is important to consider the region you want to work in.
  - Do you want to be living at home? Do you want to stay in the same city as your university? Do you need to support a family? Are you someone who enjoys living in rural versus coastal areas?
  - Speak to family and friends to aid and advise you.
  - Speak to older dental colleagues to give you further information about regions within the United Kingdom.

The list below gives the schemes that are available for DF1 applications. They may be subject to change in the forthcoming year. The HE region or deanery is displayed in **bold** and scheme names are displayed below them. A virtual map of DF1 schemes in the United Kingdom may be found at https://maps.google.co .uk/maps/ms?msid=209915530480942479969.0004c3c6972fd1afc3248&msa=0 (accessed 13 November 2015).

HE East Midlands
  Chesterfield Scheme
  Leicester Scheme
  Lincoln Scheme
  Loughborough Scheme
  Northampton Scheme
  Nottingham Scheme

HE East of England
  Basildon Scheme

Bedford Scheme
Essex Coast Scheme
Ipswich Scheme
Norwich Scheme
Peterborough Scheme
Welwyn Garden City Scheme

HE Kent, Surrey and Sussex
Central Scheme
Coastal Scheme
East Scheme
South Scheme
West Scheme

HE North East
GPT Scheme
North 1 Scheme
North 2 Scheme
South 1 Scheme
South 2 Scheme
West Scheme

HE North West
Blackburn Scheme
Lancaster Scheme
North Manchester Scheme
Pennine Scheme
Wythenshawe Scheme

HE North West (Mersey)
Aintree Scheme
Chester Scheme
Clatterbridge Scheme
Speke Scheme

HE South West
Bath Scheme
Bristol Scheme
Exeter Scheme
Plymouth Scheme
Salisbury Scheme
Taunton Scheme
Truro Scheme

HE Thames Valley / HE Wessex
Berkshire Scheme
Buckinghamshire / Milton Keynes Scheme

Oxfordshire Scheme
Portsmouth Scheme
Winchester Scheme
HE West Midlands
City Scheme
Coventry Scheme
Russells Hall Scheme (March only)
Solihull Scheme
Stafford Scheme
Telford Scheme
Worcester Scheme
HE Yorkshire and the Humber
East Yorkshire / North Lincolnshire Scheme
GPT Scheme
Harrogate Scheme
Sheffield and Doncaster Scheme
Wakefield and Dewsbury Scheme
York Scheme
London Shared Services
Northwick Park (March only)
Northwick Park
QMUL – Bart's Scheme
South East London Scheme
South West London Scheme
UCL– Eastman Scheme
Northern Ireland Deanery
Northern Ireland Scheme (August only)
Wales Deanery
East Wales Scheme
Glamorgan Scheme
North Wales Scheme
South Wales Scheme
South West Wales Scheme
Port Talbot Scheme

DF1 interview – format

Assessments are scheduled to take place in late November in six centres across the United Kingdom.

INTERVIEW TIPS

✓ Read all emails sent by the examining body prior to the interview date thoroughly and clearly, as they outline the majority of what is needed on the day, where the interview is and so forth. Do not discard them.

✓ Print out all relevant documents received.

✓ Compile all relevant documents and extras needed for the day – for example, bank statement, passport pictures.

✓ Work out the most efficient route to your interview.

✓ Top up Oyster cards or fill up with petrol beforehand.

✓ Dress smartly – boys: simple suit; girls: simple suit, long dresses or skirts and blouses.

✓ Girls – keep makeup simple.

✓ Keep a clear mind – do not plan other errands or have your mind elsewhere.

✓ Be confident!

✓ Speak clearly, comprehensively and steadily.

✓ Do not guess or make up answers; it is better to state 'I do not know'.

✓ Once it is over do not dwell!

The assessment process consists of:

1 Professional, leadership and management skills – objective structured clinical examination (OSCE) station. (10 minutes)
2 Clinical communication skills – OSCE station with real actors. (10 minutes)
3 Situational judgment test (SJT) – 56 SJT questions comprising both ranking-based SJTs and 'best of three' SJTs (105 minutes, discussed further in Chapter 3).

Professionalism, management and leadership skills station

This station is more like a mini viva station with the candidate discussing the scenario with two assessors. The candidate will be given a mark by both assessors, who will then collate their marks to calculate an average score for the student. Candidates will have 5 minutes to prepare in advance and 10 minutes for the actual station. (See mark scheme template in Chapter 3.)

Clinical communication skills station

This station will consist of a typical patient-dentist role-play scenario where an actor will be posing as the patient with a clinical problem. There will also be an assessor in the room, although he will have no involvement in the role play. The candidate will be marked by both the assessor and the actor in the role play (see mark scheme template in Chapter 3). Candidates will have 5 minutes to prepare for the station by reading and familiarizing themselves with the scenario and then 10 minutes for the actual station.

Scotland applications

Scotland has its own application process for which all year-five students can apply. The application for Scotland closes in early January and is done by emailing dental.recruitment@nes.scot.nhs.uk.

There is an application form to complete and to send to dental recruitment for Scotland. Supporting documentation is needed, such as proof of identity – one copy of photographic ID and two copies of confirmation of address.

CHAPTER 3

The SJT exam

What is an SJT?

The situational judgement test exam is designed to assess nonacademic skills and ethical values rather than clinical skills. Situational judgement tests are a measurement method designed to assess an individual's judgement regarding situations in day-to-day working practice. These questions provide an effective method of assessing the key attributes required in dentistry:
- professional qualities;
- coping with pressure;
- communicating effectively;
- teamwork;
- putting patients' interests first.

Format of the exam

The exam consists of 56 SJT questions comprising both ranking-based SJTs and 'best of three' SJTs. Six of the SJT questions will be used for evaluation purposes. The candidate will have 105 minutes for the exam, which is machine marked.

The Dental Foundation Interview Guide: with Situational Judgement Tests, First Edition.
Zahid Siddique, Shivana Anand and Helena Lewis-Greene.
© 2017 John Wiley & Sons, Ltd. Published 2017 by John Wiley & Sons, Ltd.

Ranking-based SJTs

Candidates will be given a question with five possible responses to specific situations. They will then need to rank the five options from the most to least appropriate usually from A to E.

'Best of three' SJTs

The candidate will be presented with a situation question in which there will be eight possible answers. The candidate will then need to choose the **three most appropriate answers when all of the answers are considered together.**

Marking format of the exam

Ranking-based SJTs

As explained above, the candidate is asked to rank five possible answers from the most appropriate to the least appropriate. The table below demonstrates how the candidate can score the maximum mark of 20 points for each question.

For example, if the answer to a question is ACBDE, with A being the most appropriate and E being the least appropriate, your score will be calculated according to a matrix which can look like the one in Table 3.1. Ranking the options correctly scores the candidate 20 marks.

Best of three SJTs

In this format the candidate must choose the three most suitable options when all the options are considered together. Each option scores four marks and therefore a maximum of 12 marks can be scored for each question. For example, if the correct three options are BCD the candidate will score 12 marks for choosing BCD, eight marks for only choosing two correct options, for example BCA, and four marks if the candidate only chose one correct option, for example BAE.

Table 3.1 Mark scheme for ranking-based SJTs.

Correct ranking	If you ranked it first	If you ranked it second	If you ranked it third	If you ranked it fourth	If you ranked it fifth
A	4	3	2	1	0
C	3	4	3	2	1
B	2	3	4	3	2
D	1	2	3	4	3
E	0	1	2	3	4

CHAPTER 4

Definitions and legalities

Definitions

General Dental Council

The GDC is the primary regulator of dental professionals, with a principal role in ensuring patient safety. There are 12 members on the GDC; six are dentists and six are lay people. The functions of the GDC are to maintain the dental register, to ensure quality, to supervise dental education and to administer any disciplinary action required against its members where appropriate. Section 38 of the Dentists Act states that it is illegal to practise without being placed on the GDC register.

Care Quality Commission (CQC)

The CQC has been checking that healthcare service providers are meeting national standards for safe, effective, compassionate and high-quality care since 1 April 2009. It encourages all healthcare employers to always make continual improvements. The CQC hold inspections with all practices that should be registered with the CQC.

Faculty of General Dental Practitioners (FGDP)

Formed in 1992 as the academic home for general dental practitioners (GDPs). The FGDP(UK) is based at the Royal College of Surgeons of England (RCSEng) and aims to improve the standard of care delivered to patients through standard setting, publications, postgraduate training and assessment, continuing professional development, education and research.

The Dental Foundation Interview Guide: with Situational Judgement Tests, First Edition.
Zahid Siddique, Shivana Anand and Helena Lewis-Greene.
© 2017 John Wiley & Sons, Ltd. Published 2017 by John Wiley & Sons, Ltd.

Clinical commissioning groups

These are overseen by NHS England and are grouped in geographical areas by commissioning healthcare services including general practitioners, hospitals, dental services, pharmacists and specialist services.

Local authority teams

Local authority teams deal with practical, operational and administrative matters in communities. They report back to the NHS commissioning board. They have replaced primary care trusts (PCTs) but work with a central policy and consistent guidelines.

Clinical governance

Clinical governance is a systematic approach to maintaining and improving the quality of patient care within a health system such as the NHS. NHS organizations have a duty to seek quality improvement, maintain quality healthcare and minimize risks. The practice framework is subdivided into 12 distinct areas.

Indemnity provider

This is an organization to support and provide impartial confidential advice to dental professionals. The majority of indemnity providers are nonprofit organizations. It is a legal requirement for dentists to have in place arrangements for compensation to be arranged if they cause harm. A sum is paid on behalf of the dentists for the loss experienced by patients.

National Institute for Health and Care Excellence (NICE)

The NICE publishes guidelines in:
- health technology within the NHS;
- clinical practice;
- public health sector workers in healthcare.
  Examples of clinical practice include:
- Prescription of antibiotics. The guidelines changed in 2008, so no prophylaxis against infective endocarditis is given. Advise patients against cover and liaise with their cardiologist for further assistance if needed.
- Extraction of wisdom teeth:
  - unrestorable caries;
  - no treatment of pulpal and PA pathology are available;
  - cellulitis;
  - abscess;
  - osteomyelitis;
  - internal and external resorption on wisdom teeth or the adjacent tooth;

- fracture;
- disease of follicle – cyst/tumour;
- reconstructive surgery;
- in field of tumour resection;
- pericoronitis for more than 2 years, one severe.
- Bisphosphonates – can cause bisphosphonate related osteonecrosis of the jaw (BRONJ). If a patient is on IV or oral bisphosphonates for more than 2 years, this may be a contraindication for extractions.

Legislation for the dental team

The law related to confidentiality
Data Protection Act 1998:
- data should be processed lawfully and fairly;
- data should be processed for specific purposes;
- adequate, relevant but not excessive note keeping;
- accurate, up-to-date records – for example, medical histories;
- medical records not kept longer than necessary – 11 years or 25 years if the patient is under 18 years old;
- data should be processed in line with subject rights;
- security: passwords and locked, encrypted USB safe sticks;
- data should not be transferred to countries outside EEA without adequate protection.

Freedom of Information Act 2000:
- the patient has a right to access notes and records;
- the dentist has to give copy within 40 days of receipt of request;
- radiographs are the dentist's property;
- patients have the right to correct factual errors in their medical notes;
- dentists may charge a fee for radiographs: £50 for a hard copy, £10 for a digital copy.

Legislation relevant to raising concerns
Public Interest Disclosure Act (PIDA) 1998:
- A healthcare professional can break confidentiality and raise a concern if it is in the interest of the public. Qualified disclosure can occur when the law has been broken.
- Confidentiality can be broken when there is a miscarriage of justice, environmental harm, when a crime has been committed, or when there is a serious health and safety issue.
- The breach in confidentiality must be raised in good faith and undertaken using the correct process.

The law relevant to putting the patient's best interest first

- Ionising Radiation Regulations (IRR)
- Ionising Radiation (Medical Exposure) Regulations (IRMER)
- Health Technical Memorandum HTM01-05
- Publications of the Health and Safety Executive (HSE)
- Disposal of Hazardous Waste/COSHH
- Human Rights Act 1998

The law relevant to consent

Fraser guidelines

- Gillick competency and Fraser guidelines refer to the competence of a child under the age of 16 to consent to his or her own medical care. The Fraser guidelines require healthcare professionals to assume that everyone has the capacity to consent until proven otherwise. A child is someone under the age of 18 years old. Persons who usually consent for those under 18 years of age are their mother and father (as named on the child's birth certificate) if the time of birth was after 2003, or the father at time of birth if this occurred before 2003. Therefore healthcare professionals can deem people under 18 years Fraser competent until otherwise proven. 'Capacity' is assessed by giving patients information and ensuring they are able to understand, retain, weigh up the options and communicate back a decision.

Legislation relevant to consent

Mental Capacity Act 2005

- This enables those who are over 16 and lack capacity to be protected and empowered to make their own decisions. People who may lack capacity include those who have dementia, strokes, mental health issues, or learning disabilities. Healthcare professionals must assume that all have capacity until proven otherwise. They should help individuals make informed decisions themselves, assess periods of capacity versus no capacity and, if someone lacks capacity, help a decision to be made in that person's best interest.
- Decisions made should be least restrictive of the affected person's basic rights.
- The Mental Capacity Act allows for an 'independent advocate' or person provided to support decision making especially if it may significantly restrict the affected person's wellbeing.
- How should professionals assess capacity? Does the person have a severe impairment? Does the impairment cause significant issues in specific decision making?
- Capacity must be rechecked each time as there may be periods of lack of capacity interspersed with periods of capacity.
- How should professionals test for capacity? Understand the information relevant to the decision. Retain the information. Use and weigh up the information. Communicate that decision back.

Healthcare professionals must support decision making by thinking about the following:

- Has all relevant information been given?
- Could information be presented more easily?
- Have all alternatives been considered?
- Can others help with communication?
- Can the decision be delayed?
- Can decisions be made at better times during the day or in better environments?
- Have other methods of communication been explored?

Those who can help with decision making include:

- guardians;
- those previous named by the patient;
- those who take an interest in their welfare;
- those granted lasting power of attorney;
- those granted enduring power of attorney;
- a deputy appointed by Court of Protection.

Those granted a lasting power of attorney or an enduring power of attorney must make sure that the Mental Capacity Act statutory principles are followed if the patient does not have the capacity to make decisions. Enduring power of attorneys are valid from before date when the Mental Capacity Act came into force (1 October 2007).

All members registered with the GDC must have training in the Mental Capacity Act.

Clinical governance

NHS organizations have a duty to seek quality improvements, maintain quality healthcare and minimize risks. Clinical governance has seven pillars:

1 Clinical effectiveness
2 Audit and peer review
3 Risk management
4 Education
5 Patient information and safety
6 Using information and IT
7 Staff training.

Risk factors may be minimized by:

1 Identifying the risk
2 Assessing the risk
3 Removing the risk factors
4 Reducing the risk factors
5 Weighing up the outcome

6 Sending adverse incident reports and significant event auditing to the National Patient Safety Agency (NPSA).

The clinical governance framework is subdivided into 12 distinct areas, which are listed below.

Infection control

Supporting document HTM 01-05 – *Decontamination in Primary-Care Dental Practices*:

- this is an essential requirement for best practice;
- it requires involvement of the whole dental team: adequate staff training needed for CPD;
- every practice should have written infection control policy which should be followed;
- procedures should be regularly monitored during clinical sessions and routinely audited;
- all members of the dental team should understand and practise procedures: regular discussions at team meetings are recommended;
- employers have responsibility to provide safe and hygienic environment for employees and patients.

Child protection and safeguarding

Supporting document: *Children and Vulnerable Adults:*

- dentists have a wider responsibility for the welfare of patients, which is not just limited to clinical care;
- all members of the dental team have a responsibility to protect patients from harm and should understand what actions need to be taken if they have any concerns;
- they should be able to recognize signs of abuse or neglect and find out about local procedures and follow them – raising concerns appropriately;
- induction and training may be needed;
- all staff need enhanced criminal record bureau (CRB) or now known as disclosure and barring service (DBS) checks;
- patient safety: all staff should be open and honest about any incidents, practice policy should be followed on what to do, there should be contemporaneous record keeping, investigations should be followed, action should be taken where appropriate, lessons should be learned and there should be reflection at a staff meetings.

   Staff should:

- listen and observe the child;
- seek an explanation from both child and parent or carer;
- retain contemporaneous records of everything seen or discussed;
- consider whether they suspect maltreatment or not;
- record all actions taken, including their professional conclusion;
- discuss concerns with colleagues, senior staff members and safeguarding lead;
- note that informal advice can be taken from local social services anonymously.

Radiography

Supporting documents: *Ionising Radiation (Medical Exposure) Regulations 2000; Health and Safety at Work Act 1974:*

- dental radiographs are taken very frequently – although the dose is small each time, professionals should always consider the collective effect;
- a radiation protection adviser and supervisor must be allocated to each practice;
- training records should be kept for all staff;
- staff should consider the justification for and authorization of radiography;
- they should consider equipment: keep maintenance records;
- quality assurance – there should be a radiography maintenance plan;
- aim for 70% grade 1 and 20% not more than grade 2.

Staff, patient, public and environmental safety

Supporting documents: *Health and Safety at Work Act 1974, Reporting of Injuries, Diseases and Dangerous Occurrences Regulations (RIDDOR) 2005.*

This section outlines all duties that employers have to their employees and the public, plus duties employees have to themselves and one another. Some of these include:

- providing necessary instruction, training and supervision and implementing health and safety practice policy;
- reporting injuries, diseases, dangerous occurrences;
- analysing procedures and initiating changes as a result;
- ensuring that all potentially harmful substances are handled and stored safely;
- providing a safe work environment;
- dealing appropriately with hazardous waste;
- disposing of mercury and amalgam correctly;
- dealing appropriately with asbestos;
- handling anaesthetic gases;
- ensuring electrical safety;
- taking fire precautions;
- handling infection control correctly;
- taking appropriate precautions regarding radiation;
- noting the dates of medicines and clinical products;
- handling storage correctly;
- keeping adequate records.

Evidence-based practice and research

Supporting documents: *NICE guidelines, Faculty of Dental Surgeons guidance:*

- follow relevant NICE guidelines – for example, with regard to recall intervals and wisdom-tooth removal;
- evidence-based practice should be reflected in treatment plans, delivering better oral health;
- this should be evident in advice given regarding caries, toothbrush use, fluoride, healthy eating, periodontal matters, smoking cessation, alcohol misuse, tooth

erosion, and crowns/cuspal coverage for endodontically treated molars;

- there should be compliance with referral protocols, for example the Index of Orthodontic Treatment Need (IOTN);
- continuing professional development (CPD) should be evidence based.

Prevention and public health

Supporting document: *Delivering Better Oral Health (DBOH)* 2014:

- evidence-based prevention policy for all oral diseases and conditions;
- delivering better oral health – smoking cessation, alcohol consumption, diet, fluoride, toothbrushing, caries, periodontal, erosion.

Clinical records, patient privacy and confidentiality

Supporting documents: *Data Protection Act 1998, Caldicott Guidelines 1997, GDC Standards: Section 4:*

- clinical records should be securely stored: locked/password protected;
- there should be compliance with relevant legislation;
- confidentiality should be maintained in all practice settings by all practice staff;
- clinical audit reports should be kept.

Staff involvement and development

- Staff recruitment: relevant qualifications, experience, skills, abilities – scope of practice.
- Pre-employment checks: immunization, Disclosure and Barring Service (DBS), registration, indemnity.
- Discrimination policy: written procedure manual including employment policies, for example regarding bullying, harassment, sickness, absence.
- Appropriate staff training: dealing with complaints, appointing someone as a main point of contact and for basic life support.
- Maintenance and CPD: CPD is a mandatory requirement and employers should ensure that staff undergo this.
- Clinical governance: quality assurance should be monitored via clinical audit and peer review. Meetings should be well attended by all staff and contributions should be made via staff feedback and surveys.
- There should be a confidential process to allow staff to raise concerns: a practice policy should be in place with an identified lead and with links to practitioners' advice and support schemes (PASS).

Clinical staff requirements and records

Supporting documents: *GDC Standards – Section 7:*

- all staff should be appropriately trained, registered and indemnified;
- staff should have up-to-date CPD;

- all staff should know and follow policies and protocol for raising concerns and handling complaints;
- staff should be aware of changes implemented as a result of any concern and investigations.

Patient information and involvement

Supporting documents: *GDC Standards – Section 1:*
- Communicating effectively: encourage questions and ensure understanding.
- Patient leaflets should be available in a variety of languages used locally.
- Patient feedback – surveys and suggestion boxes.
- Treatment plans: written and signed – there should be valid consent.
- Clear and effective complaints procedure: written, readily available and can easily lead to changes being made.

Fair and accessible care

- Access to interpreters.
- Disability adjustments: ramps, hearing loops – reasonable efforts made to accommodate disabilities.
- Emergency appointments available during the day – open-access appointments.
- All patients treated fairly.
- Audits and reports; changes made where necessary.

Clinical audit and peer review

- All staff involved in choosing audit subjects and procedure and in peer review.
- Learning outcomes, changes communicated to all staff and local primary care trust.
- All staff attend meetings and contribute.

CHAPTER 5

Important notes for revision

Standards for the dental team

These standards are from the GDC, used with permission. The information is correct at the time of going to press. Please visit the GDC website to check for any changes since publication: http://www.gdc-uk.org/Dentalprofessionals/ Standards/Documents/Standards%20for%20the%20Dental%20Team.pdf (accessed 10 November 2015).

There are nine principles that registered dental professionals must keep to at all times.

As a GDC registrant you must:

1 Put patients' interests first.
2 Communicate effectively with patients.
3 Obtain valid consent.
4 Maintain and protect patients' information.
5 Have a clear and effective complaints procedure.
6 Work with colleagues in a way that is in patients' best interests.
7 Maintain, develop and work within your professional knowledge and skills.

The Dental Foundation Interview Guide: with Situational Judgement Tests, First Edition.
Zahid Siddique, Shivana Anand and Helena Lewis-Greene.
© 2017 John Wiley & Sons, Ltd. Published 2017 by John Wiley & Sons, Ltd.

8 Raise concerns if patients are at risk.

9 Make sure your personal behaviour maintains patients' confidence in you and the dental profession.

Standards for the dental team apply to:

✓ dentists;

✓ dental nurses;

✓ dental hygienists;

✓ dental therapists;

✓ orthodontic therapists;

✓ dental technicians;

✓ clinical dental technicians.

The principles are all equally important and are not listed in order of priority. They are supplemented by additional guidance documents which can be found at www.gdc-uk.org (accessed 10 November 2015) and which you must also follow. You have an individual responsibility to behave professionally and follow these principles at all times.

The standards set out what you must do. If you do not meet these standards, you may be removed from the GDC register and will not be able to work as a dental professional.

The guidance is there to help you to meet the standards. You are expected to follow the guidance, to use your professional judgment, demonstrate insight at all times and be able to justify any decision that is not in line with the guidance. Serious or persistent failure to follow the guidance could see you removed from our register and not able to work as a dental professional.

Consent

Consent is 'permission or agreement for an action to occur'. Training must be undertaken by all dentists in order for them to take valid and comprehensive consent from individual patients. It is important to see the difference between competence and capacity.

General Dental Council standards state that professionals should:

• Obtain valid consent before starting treatment, explaining all the relevant options and the possible costs.

• Make sure that patients (or their representatives) understand the decisions they are being asked to make.

• Make sure that the patient's consent remains valid at each stage of investigation or treatment.

Competence

This is a key point to consider when dealing with consent. For patients to give valid consent they must be deemed to be 'competent'. This requires them to understand fully all the information provided to them regarding their treatment and care. Based on this information they should then have the capability to make a rational decision. Competence is a legal judgement.

Capacity

Capacity to consent is a medical judgement. Capacity is assessed formally and has to be judged by healthcare professionals in order to conclude that patients are able to understand their management, comprehend the risks and benefits, retain the information and make a decision based on all the information.

Competence and capacity have similar connotations. It is important, however, that both are assessed at the time in conjunction with the proposed care plan and each stage must state whether the patient was capable of consenting.

Professionals must comply fully with the Mental Capacity Act 2005 in all circumstances and a patient's capacity must be assessed before consent can be obtained. The four areas considered are:

- the patient must understand all information given;
- the patient must be able to retain the information;
- the patient must be able to use and weigh up the risks and benefits of the information;
- the patient must be able to communicate back a decision based on a balanced rationale.

All adults are assumed to have capacity to consent until otherwise proven. This is to ensure patients have autonomy and full control on their decisions regarding their care. Patients may refuse treatment against your advice but this does not mean that they lack capacity. Those with mental illnesses, those who cannot communicate as easily, are young or have a different belief set should not be presumed to lack capacity. Senior colleagues should always be consulted if the healthcare professional is unsure as to whether a patient lacks capacity to consent. If a patient is deemed to lack capacity then the dentist should always act in the best interest of that patient without discrimination and try to involve the patient wherever possible. It is also good practice to involve more senior experienced colleagues to provide advice on how best to treat the patient.

Seeking consent from a competent patient

There are many types of consent but, within dentistry, we are mainly concerned with three types of consent. These are:

1 Voluntary
   - Patient decides without consultation.
   - No pressure is imposed.

○ The patient can refuse treatment or withdraw at any time.

○ An example is the patient opening his or her mouth for an examination.

2 Verbal

○ The patient states verbally that he or she is happy with the procedure.

○ There is discussion regarding the risks and benefits of a proposed treatment.

○ There is continuous discussion aided by information over a period of time.

3 Informed

○ There is discussion regarding the risks and benefits of a proposed treatment.

○ There is continuous discussion aided by information over a period of time.

○ There is clear agreement on contract and charges with any amendments reconsented.

○ Example: treatment planning form FP17 – all treatment to be carried out is written on this form in language understandable to the patient. The form outlines all risks/benefits of treatment and includes both NHS and private cost of treatment. Patients keep a signed copy for themselves and the dentist keeps a signed copy in the patient's notes.

Verbal versus written consent

Contemporaneous notekeeping is of the utmost importance within dentistry. Records are taken as part of the process outlining what both parties agreed upon, including a shared vision of outcomes of treatment including risks and benefits proposed. An example of this is the official NHS FP17 treatment planning form.

Voluntary and verbal consent may be sufficient in most cases, for example when a special investigation is to be taken such as a 'tender to percussion' test or general examination. In these cases, patients must understand what the procedure is and how it will be of benefit to them. If they agree to minor procedures, verbal consent may be enough in their clinical notes.

Written consent is needed for any operative dental treatment and larger procedures. Some examples are as followed:

• complex procedures, such as surgical extractions;

• general anaesthetic;

• IV or nasal sedation

• the majority of paediatric procedures;

• when clinical care is not primarily the purpose of the procedure, for example aesthetic treatments;

• when treatment is for research;

• when clinical photography is to be taken.

Competence and capacity in children

See the section on children and vulnerable adults in this chapter, below.

Confidentiality

General Dental Council Standard 4: maintain and protect patients' information:
- Make and keep contemporaneous, complete and accurate patient records.
- Protect the confidentiality of patients' information and only use it for the purpose for which it was given.
- Only release patients' information without their permission in exceptional circumstances.
- Ensure that patients can have access to their records.
- Keep patients' information secure at all times, whether your records are held on paper or electronically.

'Maintain and protect patients' information' is one of the core ethical principles for dentists set by the GDC. The right to confidentiality is paramount in the dentist-patient relationship. This protection of information creates trust and provides the right environment and culture for patients to feel safe during their interaction with the dentist and the wider dental team. As a dentist you have both an ethical and legal duty to keep patient information confidential and patients reserve the right to keep information about them confidential under the Data Protection Act 1998. The GDC sets standards for all dentists to enable them to achieve and maintain patient confidentiality where possible. It must be noted there may be some circumstances where confidentiality may be breached and this will be discussed further below.

A breach of patient confidentiality contrary to the GDCs standards by dentists or the wider dental team could result in the dentists' fitness to practise being found impaired, leaving them liable to action being taken upon their registration.

Key facts and information regarding confidentiality

There are circumstances when patient confidentiality needs to be breached. This could be to help the patient, for example by sharing information with other healthcare professionals regarding treatment, or it may be to protect a member of the public involved with the patient. The following situations are examples of when confidentiality can be breached:

1 Disclosing information to other healthcare professionals or carers involved in the patients overall care. This could be, for example, something as simple as asking a dental colleague for a second opinion or writing a referral letter to another dentist or hospital department regarding the patient's care, or liaising with the patient's GP in providing a more holistic care approach for the patient. Breaches such as these occur routinely in practice and are accepted by patients as long as diligence is taken with the information provided, ensuring that it is limited to necessary information only. Patients are deemed to have provided implied consent and must be made fully aware each time any information is passed on to another healthcare professional. If the patient has any objections

to this, it is the professional's obligation to respect the patient's choice and try to seek the help needed for the patient without breaching confidentiality.

2 Divulging information as required by law. Information may be disclosed through a court order even if it is against the patient's wishes. If a court order has been presented then it is the professional's legal duty to comply and provide the information required.

3 Releasing information for the sake of public interest and public safety, protecting the patient or others who are at risk of harm or death in not doing so.

There are some situations where professionals will need to release confidential information to protect the patient and others, where they feel the benefit to society outweighs the duty of confidentiality to the patient. Example scenarios of such situations could include treating a neglected child or vulnerable adult. If a female patient being treated for trauma injuries reveals, during her appointment, that she is being physically abused by her partner but does not want you to inform anyone, you might feel that the patient is at serious risk of harm from her partner and feel it is in her best interest to inform other authorities such as the social services or police without gaining valid consent from the patient. It is important to consider who else may be affected by this situation, assessing the wider picture. Does the patient have any children? Could they also be victims of abuse? Is their safety and wellbeing at risk? Considering factors like these will make it easier for you to decide if patient confidentiality must be breached in order to have a greater benefit to the patient and others involved, be it family members or society generally.

Another common case is child abuse. If you deem that it is in the best interest of the patient to share information with a third party who can help with the patient's circumstances, be it a trusted family member or social service, it is important you do so promptly. It is important to remember, with cases such as child abuse, that there is a duty upon you to share information with other agencies such as social services or the police. If for any reason you decide not to report, you should be able to justify your decision fully. If you suspect a child is being abused in any way and you decide to share information with other agencies, you must still tell the child's parent or legal guardian you are doing so, unless you feel that this may put the patient at further risk of harm.

Complicated cases such as these should always be dealt with delicately, especially if you lack experience in dealing with them. In such a case it is important you seek impartial confidential advice from senior colleagues or your indemnity provider who will be able to assist and guide you.

Keeping the patient informed

In any situation where you need to breach confidentiality it is essential that you discuss it with the patient first, gaining consent and informing the patient of your reasons for disclosure. This may prove to be a difficult conversation; however, reassuring the patient you are doing it in his or her interest or for a greater benefit will make it easier for the patient to understand. If a situation arises where you breach confidentiality without notifying the patient because you feel that by informing the patient of the breach it may cause further harm and risk to the either the patient or someone else, it is important that you gain advice from your union and other senior colleagues who may be able to help before disclosing any information.

Complaints

A complaint is any expression of dissatisfaction by a patient or a patient's representative about a dental service or treatment, whether justified or not. Most complaints arise after a series of smaller events are experienced, which leave the patient feeling disappointed. A triggering factor can lead to a complaint. Most complaints arise primarily because a patient's expectation are not met or accounted for.

GDC Standard 5 – 'Have a clear and effective complaints procedure'

The complaint may be justified or not, spoken or written and about any part of the service delivered. Handling the complaints well maintains and improves the rapport and relationship with your patient, hopefully preventing more complaints. Most complaints are about communication, so handling the complaint clearly and effectively aids ease of outcome.

All practices must have a complaints-handling procedure for patients and staff members to follow:

✓ it must be visible;

✓ it should allow complaints to be addressed speedily;

✓ it should allow complaints to be investigated fully and fairly;

✓ it should respect confidentiality;

✓ it should be clearly written;

✓ there should be no dental jargon;

✓ it should clearly explain outcomes;

✓ it should lead to improved service.

Setting the framework
- Patients should know who to contact.
- Practice employees should familiarize themselves with complaints procedures.
- Practice employees should have appropriate training.

The complaints procedure
1 Acknowledge the complaint and provide the patient with the practice complaint procedure.

2 Inform the dental defence organization if you require advice.

3 Inform the patients of timescales and stages involved.

4 Acknowledge the complaint in writing, by email or by telephone as soon as you receive it – 3 working days maximum but ideally within 24 hours.

5 Respond to the complaint within 10 days – if circumstances arise that prevent this, ensure that the patient is aware of different timescales ensuring you regularly update him or her (at least every 10 working days).

6 Hold a staff meeting for peer review, audit and feedback on the outcome of the complaint.

Dealing with the complaints

- Do not be defensive – use the REACH approach (see box).
- Deal with all complaints and offer appropriate solutions within an accepted timeframe.
- Offer an apology – saying sorry shows concern, understanding and empathy, it does not mean you are admitting any responsibility.
- If justified, offer compensation.
- After investigation: send a letter – detailing what has been decided, practical solutions, compensation (if justified).
- If the patient is still not satisfied, forward the patient's complaint to NHS Complaints Procedure Services (CPS), the Dental Complaints Service (DCS) (for private practices) or the Patient Advice Liaison Services (PALS) (hospitals).
- An Ombudsman can be asked to investigate a complaint by a patient formally at any time.

R – Recognition

E – Empathise

A – Apologize

C – Compensation

H – Honesty

Scope of practice

General Dental Council registered dental care professionals are:

1 Dentists.

2 Dental nurses.

3 Dental hygienists.

4 Dental therapists.

5 Dental technicians.

6 Clinical dental technicians.

7 Orthodontic therapists.

'Scope of practice' guidelines from the GDC give a comprehensive list of what each DCP (dental care professional) can and cannot do. The standards set by the GDC state that all DCPs must:

- work effectively;
- have appropriate support – especially in medical emergencies;
- delegate and refer patients when not competent and only accept patients if competent;
- communicate clearly;
- manage and lead the team using everyone's skill set.
  When referring patients:
- clearly request all appropriate information;
- gain valid consent;
- if consent is received – be clear and competent and share information;
- know when to refer;
- explain the process to the patient;
- clear contemporaneous record keeping.

Continued professional development (CPD)

General Dental Council standard 7: 'maintain, develop and work within your professional knowledge and skills'

All members of the dental team must comply in carrying out verifiable and nonverifiable CPD on a 5-year rota. All members must work within their scope, develop their professional evidence-based practice and comply with the guidance from authorities such as NICE, FGDP. Continued professional development upholds the GDC standard of maintaining, developing and working within your professional knowledge and skills.

Foundation dentist trainees have their CPD cycle start in the January of their foundation year. It is important to keep a log of CPD, electronic personal development plans (ePDPs) and any additional courses attended for their CPD log.

Dentist = 250 hours total CPD, of which verifiable CPD = 75 hours.
✓ Medical emergencies = 10 hours.

✓ Infection control = 5 hours.

✓ Radiography and radiation protection =5 hours.
Nurse = 150 hours total CPD of which verifiable CPD = 50 hours.
✓ Medical emergencies = 10 hours.

✓ Infection control = 5 hours.

✓ Radiography and radiation protection = 5 hours.

Other CPD themes include:
- legal considerations and ethics;
- dental materials – technicians can use this instead of 'radiography and radiation protection' as verifiable continuing professional development (vCPD);
- photography;
- business;
- complaints handling;
- techniques;
- oral medicine;
- periodontology.

Online personal development plan (ePDP)

An ePDP is an online log-in book of reflection and analysis on your dental experiences.

Audit

Local teams have a list of possible audit projects. Practices can also choose a project or reaudit to compare and contrast results over a period of time. Audit can be accepted as vCPD. It should include:
- aims and objectives;
- a summary of methodology;
- a timetable;
- detailed educational source material.

Peer review

Four to eight dentists discuss clinical governance, safeguarding and best practice, which includes clinical and administrative matters. The organizer must dictate frequency of meetings, venue and proposed review titles and can submit these to the local scheme.

Raising concerns

GDC standard 8: 'raise concerns if patients are at risk'

Raising concerns is different from making a complaint. A complaint must prove a case with appropriate evidence. When raising a concern you should not be expected to prove the malpractice but you are opening a discussion with the aim of acting in the patient's best interest. All practices should have a policy about raising concerns, with which all staff members should familiarize themselves.

A concern must be raised if the patient might be at risk due to:
- The health, behaviour or professional performance of a colleague – unprofessional behaviour is unacceptable and should be acted upon.
- Any aspect of the environment where treatment is provided.

- Someone asking you to do something that you think conflicts with your duties to put patients' interests first and/or to act to protect them.

Concerns may be raised with:

- senior colleagues;
- the lead person for raising concerns;
- employers;
- dental defence organization;
- professional associations;
- Public Concern at Work;
- Care Quality Commission;
- General Dental Council.

There should be an open policy for raising concerns. Staff should feel encouraged and confident in doing this, there should be a clear and efficient system in place for it and staff should feel supported after raising a concern. If further guidance is needed this can be taken from the Public Disclosure Act 1998 (PIDA), which protects employees who raise genuine concerns in the NHS and privately.

The process for raising concerns

1 Keep a log book of the series of events including email threads, time and dates of events and any colleagues' opinions on the matter.
2 Familiarize yourself with the practice policy for raising concerns.
3 You can take informal advice from your defence organization at any point throughout the raising concerns journey.
4 Approach the raising concerns lead, practice manager or employer regarding your concern.
5 Try to solve the concern within the practice. If this is not applicable then approach your local primary care organization or NHS hospital trust.
6 Refer the matter to the GDC if:
   - it is not practical to raise a concern at the local level;
   - the local level has failed;
   - serious problems have occurred: indecency, violence, crime, illegal practice, victimization or a cover up.

Child protection and vulnerable adults

All GDC registrants must raise concerns about the possible abuse of children or vulnerable adults. The standards for the dental team state:

> … You must raise any concerns you may have about the possible abuse or neglect of children or vulnerable adults. You must know who to contact for further advice and how to refer concerns to an appropriate authority such as your local social services department.

... You must find out about local procedures for the protection of children and vulnerable adults. You must follow these procedures if you suspect that a child or vulnerable adult might be at risk because of abuse or neglect.

In the United Kingdom, a child is anyone under the age of 18. Once children reach the age of 16 they are presumed by law to be competent and their confidentiality must be respected as if they were adults. With regard to healthcare, children aged 16–17 cannot refuse treatment that is in their best interest if it has been agreed by a person with parental responsibility or by a court order. Conversely, parents or legal guardians cannot overrule the decision of a competent child aged 16–17 when what the parents/guardian want is not in the best interest of the child. In practice, however, at times it can be very difficult to start/complete a treatment that has been consented by a parent if the child in the chair is not willing to cooperate. In such cases it is important to not force the treatment on the child as this may make the experience worse for the child. The professional should think of alternative routes for treatment such as secondary care referrals.

Children under 16 are not to be assumed to have the capacity to consent; hence, a parent (named on the child's birth certificate) must be present to advocate any dental treatment required. Children under the age of 16 are allowed to give valid consent only if they are deemed Gillick or Fraser competent. Gillick or Fraser competency applies to children who have a sufficient understanding and maturity to enable them to understand fully what treatment is proposed including weighing up all risks and benefits of treatment and communicating back decisions based on all the information provided to them.

A 'vulnerable adult' is 'a person above the age of 18 years who is or may be in need of community care services (including healthcare) by reason of mental or other disability, age or illness; and who is unable to take care of him or herself, or unable to protect him or herself against significant harm or exploitation.'

Spotting the first signs of abuse

A dental professional is likely to notice injuries to the head and neck region and also to the teeth in conjunction with welfare concerns. Signs and symptoms may include:
- bruising;
- burns;
- lip grazes;
- bite marks;
- eye injuries.

Most of these injuries may not be coincident with the tooth injury and fall into the 'zone of protection' The triangle of safety must be carefully assessed, clinical considerations made, expert guidance taken and all factors must be taken into consideration.

There are four types of abuse:
1 Sexual.

2 Mental.

3 Physical.

4 Neglect.

Neglect includes frequent caries, plaque stagnation and unclean clothing, which are all aspects that professionals can very easily assess in the dental room. If you make a professional judgement and decide not to share your concern with the appropriate authority, you must be able to justify how you came to this decision. You should contact your defence organization for advice.

For more information on child protection and health, see the following web site: http://www.cpdt.org.uk/data/files/Resources/Childprotectionandthedentalteam_ v1_4_Nov09.pdf (accessed 10 November 2015).

A checklist of sources to consult during revision

- ☐ GDC Standards for the Dental Team
- ☐ Raising Concerns
- ☐ Dental Team Working
- ☐ Scope of Practice
- ☐ Direct Access
- ☐ Consent
- ☐ Complaints
- ☐ Confidentiality
- ☐ NICE Guidelines
  - ☐ Steroid Cover
  - ☐ Extraction of 8s
  - ☐ Antibiotic Prophylaxis
  - ☐ Bisphisphonates
  - ☐ Conscious Sedation
  - ☐ General Anaesthetic
- ☐ Delivering Better Oral Health
- ☐ Pilot Schemes and Clinical Care Pathway
- ☐ Whitening Legislation and Bleaching
- ☐ CQC, COSHH
- ☐ Clinical Governance
  - ☐ Patient Information and Involvement
  - ☐ Safeguarding Children and Vulnerable Adults
  - ☐ Infection Control
  - ☐ Dental Radiography
  - ☐ Staff, Patient, Public, Environmental Safety
  - ☐ Evidence Based Practice and Research
  - ☐ Prevention and Public Health
  - ☐ Clinical Records, Patient Privacy and Confidentiality
  - ☐ Staff Involvement and Development

☐ Clinical Staff Requirements and Development
☐ Fair and Accessible Care
☐ Clinical Audit and Peer Review
☐ Quality Assurance
☐ Medical Emergency and Resus Guidelines
☐ Articles
  ☐ Breaking bad news
  ☐ Developing the dental team
  ☐ The first five years
  ☐ Drug prescriptions
  ☐ SJT
  ☐ Social media and the GDC
  ☐ Reporting criminal convictions and the GDC
  ☐ Dental protection: ethics
☐ Acts and regulations
  ☐ Data Protection Act 1998
  ☐ Employment Act 2008
  ☐ Human Rights Act 1998
  ☐ Equality Act 2010
  ☐ Public Interest Disclosure Act 1998
  ☐ Mental Capacity 2005
  ☐ Ionising Radiations Regulations (IRR) 1999
  ☐ Ionising Radiation (Medical Exposure) Regulations (IRMER) 2000
☐ Dental Organizations and Bodies
  ☐ General Dental Council (GDC)
  ☐ Faculty of General Dental Practice (FGDP)
  ☐ British Dental Association (BDA)
  ☐ Care Quality Commission (CQC)
  ☐ Dental Protection/Dental Defence Union (DDU)

CHAPTER 6

Practice scenarios

Introduction

These are scenarios. Information was correct at the time of going to press. Please visit the GDC web site to check for any changes since publication: www.gdc-uk .org (accessed 10 November 2015).

The SJTs in this book were verified and standardized by a group of dentists.

Each scenario within general practice, hospital, in a dental foundation year or any other field, will be extremely specific to the individual case. It is important to follow all necessary guidelines, referring to documents, acting logically and methodically and speaking to relevant bodies or team members throughout.

The following scenarios relate to each one of the GDC guidelines. Each scenario should be used as guidance only in understanding the basis of answering professionalism, management and leadership questions. There are guidance notes attached for all scenarios to give you a basic understanding of how to manage the scenario as a whole.

The Dental Foundation Interview Guide: with Situational Judgement Tests, First Edition.
Zahid Siddique, Shivana Anand and Helena Lewis-Greene.
© 2017 John Wiley & Sons, Ltd. Published 2017 by John Wiley & Sons, Ltd.

Professionalism, leadership and management scenarios

GDC Standard: 1. Put patients' interests first

Scenario: You see an 8-year-old boy for a new patient examination. He attends with his mother who seems uninterested. The patient looks unkempt, withdrawn and, on investigation, has multiple carious lesions and abscesses. After delivering oral-health instruction and trying to explain the plan to both mother and patient, the mother shouts aggressively at the child exclaiming this is his entire fault. You are concerned and worried about the wellbeing of this child.

What are the clinical governance issues?

How would you manage this scenario?

How can you and the team learn from this?

What are the clinical governance issues?

Dento-legal issues:

- putting patients' interests first;
- communication;
- consent;
- confidentiality;
- teamwork;
- core professional development;
- raising concerns;
- personal behaviour control.

Other clinical governance issues:

- health and safety;
- record keeping;
- child and vulnerable adult protection;
- evidence-based practice;
- prevention;
- staff training and involvement;
- clinical effectiveness;
- patient information and involvement;
- quality assurance and self-assessment (audit, peer review).

What would you do at this appointment?

Firstly, ensure the patient's best interest is put first. Even though the patient is a minor, all considerations need to be made to ensure complete safety for the patient.

Communicate effectively with the wider team. In practice there will always be someone to go to but the first port of call will be to raise concerns with the practice safeguarding lead.

You have a professional duty to explain all outcomes of the dental assessment to the patient and mother:

- explain all caries tooth by tooth;
- explain aetiology of the caries – poor diet, poor oral hygiene, neglect;
- explain the abscesses – show them to the mother in the child's mouth and on the radiographs;
- write down all the risks and benefits of treatment options;
- explain treatment options.

Try to diffuse the situation by explaining that this is now a health-and-safety issue. Explain to the mother what steps you will take – for example, that you will be speaking to the practice safeguarding lead and introduce any senior members of clinical staff, starting with your educational supervisor, to gain a second opinion.

Even though the patient is at risk, these matters must be dealt with professionally and you should try to follow consent and confidentiality procedures here.

Take a multidisciplinary approach including involving your educational supervisor or senior dentist in the practice, the patient's GP, social services and any other healthcare providers – working as a team is imperative.

Once the meeting is over and any social workers have attended, make contemporaneous notes, explicitly noting all discussions, conversations, witnesses and outcomes – all notes should be dated, timed and signed.

How can you and the team learn from this?

The health-and-safety issues raised here need to be highlighted – all practices should have a protocol for health and safety, safeguarding, child protection and team work and these should be maintained and updated regularly.

Staff training and involvement should be maintained with regular CPD in all aspects of raising a concern and child protection.

Information leaflets should be left in the practice for all patients to be aware of issues.

In this instance, an incident report form should be completed regarding the appointment and all the events that followed. The notes need to be contemporaneous and up to date on the computer system. There should be a practice incident book or folder in which the report form should be stored – a copy of this can also be attached to the patient's file.

Moving forward, regular audits should be encouraged – compare, contrast safeguarding issues, audit the practice procedure sheet, the child protection lead should be audited for consistency and outcomes should be monitored.

At the next staff meeting a peer review on the management of the appointment and any future outcomes should be discussed and noted. This allows the team to address and learn from the situation and seek further training.

GDC Standard: 2. Communicate effectively with patients

Scenario: A colleague's patient comes to practice complaining of pain for LL6. The colleague had performed endodontic treatment on this tooth. A postoperative radiograph shows a broken file in one of the canals. This has not been documented in the radiographic report and the patient was unaware of this. How would you deal with this situation?

What are the clinical governance issues here?

How would you manage this situation?

What future plans could be made to minimize risk?

What are the clinical governance issues here?

Dento-legal issues:

- ∘ acting in the patient's best interest;
- ∘ communication;
- ∘ consent;
- ∘ raising concerns;
- ∘ complaints.

Other clinical governance issues:

- ∘ evidence-based practice;
- ∘ staff training and involvement;
- ∘ clinical effectiveness;
- ∘ record keeping;
- ∘ health and safety;
- ∘ CPD, audit, peer review.

How would you manage this situation?

Your duty of care is to the patient, not the colleague. You must explain your findings to the patient. An apology will do much to alleviate the concern of the patient. Inform the patient that you will discuss the situation with the colleague who treated her initially.

If you do not feel comfortable approaching the colleague directly then discuss the issue with the practice manager, a senior member of staff or the practice principal.

A follow-up letter to the patient reassuring them that the practice will do everything possible to resolve the situation would be advisable.

Offer a consultation to a specialist endodontist (to be paid for by the practice / treating colleague). Medico legally, if the risks of file separation have not been documented, the full cost of the endodontic treatment should be paid for by the practice / treating colleague otherwise there may be other serious implications.

If the patient wants to complain, ensure you direct her to the complaints procedure. The patient can contact NHS complaints or Ombudsman if this complaint cannot be rectified locally. All complaints should be rectified locally before going to the primary care trust or General Dental Council.

Contact your indemnity provider for advice.

What future plans could be made to minimize risk?

Quality assurance needs to be reassessed. Ensure all Care Quality Commission (CQC) outcomes have policies within the practice. The CQC is responsible for ensuring that all healthcare providers are of a gold standard. They will want to see policies that address any adverse incident that might occur, who the leaders for safeguarding and raising concern are within the practice and what standard protocols are in place to deal with the day-to-day running of the practice – for example, complaints, infection control, disposal of materials, staff CPD.

All staff should have appropriate training when it comes to communication, raising concerns and complaint handling.

There should be a risk assessment of the practice. Are files being used appropriately? Are clinicians having proper training in endodontics and keeping CPD relevant? Is there a proper consent protocol? Have notes been made sufficiently, including all risks of treatment for all patients? Patient leaflets could be made to help patients to understand difficult treatments.

There should be self-assessment – audit, peer review, reaudit and comparing to other clinicians, reflection in ePDP (an online professional development plan where professionals are able to reflect, compare, contrast and state how they will better their learning).

Raise the concern with the treating colleague – follow the raising concerns guideline, speak to the raising concerns lead in the practice.

GDC Standard: 3. Obtain valid consent

Scenario: Mrs Jones attends your surgery and after assessment you decide she needs several of her teeth extracted. She suffers from Alzheimer's disease and has attended with her carer and friend. What are the issues here and what would you do next?

What are the clinical governance issues here?

How would you manage this situation?

What are the future implications for managing risk?

What are the clinical governance issues here?

Dento-legal issues:

- consent;
- putting patients' interests first;
- communication;
- confidentiality;
- teamwork.

Other clinical governance issues:

- record keeping;
- child and vulnerable adult protection;

- evidence-based practice;
- prevention;
- staff training and involvement;
- clinical effectiveness;
- patient information and involvement;
- accessibility;
- quality assurance and self-assessment (audit, peer review, patient feedback).

How would you manage this scenario?

First and foremost you must assess that Mrs Jones has capacity to make valid consent. Ensure that all options have been given to the patient to make a valid decision – leaflets, information videos, several appointments, times.

Assessing a patient's capacity includes giving the patient information, allowing the patient to retain the information, weighing up decisions and relaying the information back.

The principles of the Mental Capacity Act 2005 are:

1 A person must be assumed to have capacity unless it is established that he lacks capacity.
2 A person is not to be treated as unable to make a decision unless all practicable steps to help him to do so have been taken without success.
3 A person is not to be treated as unable to make a decision merely because he makes an unwise decision.
4 An act done, or decision made, under this Act for or on behalf of a person who lacks capacity must be done, or made, in his best interests.
5 Before the act is done, or the decision made, regard must be had to whether the purpose for which it is needed can be as effectively achieved in a way that is less restrictive of the person's rights and freedom of action.

If Mrs Jones does not have capacity to make an informed decision it is advisable that two healthcare professionals agree on this before continuing treatment.

If she has been deemed unable to consent then it is important to find out who has power of attorney, and if a legal guardian or an appointed member has been allowed to make the decisions on her behalf. If there is no kin, attorney and so forth, does she need an independent mental capacity advocate (IMCA) before treatment may be carried out?.

All decisions need to be made in the patient's best interest with all benefits outweighing the risks in order to treat.

Treatment must be the least restrictive – the option that is least likely to impair function for the patient and should include full patient cooperation and appropriate maintenance.

The full team is expected to be a part of treatment, with a multidisciplinary approach with neighbouring specialities, for example special care and sedation units. General practitioners will provide an updated medical history and any changes to dental treatment can be advised accordingly by GPs.

Clinical effectiveness is vital, especially as long duration of appointments or appointments scheduled at inappropriate timings may affect the patients cooperation and the extent to which she can be assessed. Towards the end of the day the patient's memory may deteriorate or cooperation may be reduced.

Evidence-based practice must be carried out at all times ensuring all relevant guidelines are met and any medications the patient may be taking are documented.

All records of options given, opinions and treatments not done must be justified in contemporaneous notes. Any letters between GPs, surgeons or anyone else involved in the care of the patient must be kept with records. If at any point treatment becomes out of your scope, the relevant person is to be contacted.

What are the future implications for managing risk?

Quality assurance needs to be reassessed. Ensure all CQC outcomes have policies within the practice. Ensure all staff have appropriate training when it comes to communication, raising concerns and updating their knowledge on capacity assessment and consent. All professionals should be aware of the relevant legislation.

There should be risk assessment of the practice to ensure appropriate accessibility. Are patient leaflets available? Are clinicians having proper training in treatment of vulnerable adults and keeping CPD relevant?

Is there a proper consent protocol? Have notes been made sufficiently and including proper documentation of all risks of treatment for all patients?

There should also be self-assessment – audit, peer review, reaudit, comparison to other clinicians, and reflection in the ePDP.

Raise the concern with the treating colleague – follow the raising concerns guideline, speak to the raising concerns lead in the practice.

Patient feedback will always aid in future treatment planning.

GDC Standard: 4. Maintain and protect patients' information

Scenario: You have referred an elderly patient to hospital with a persistent mouth ulcer. You suspect oral cancer. The family asks you not to inform the patient if the results of any investigations confirm diagnosis of cancer.

What are the clinical governance issues here?

How would you handle this scenario?

What are the future implications for managing risk?

What are the clinical governance issues?

Dento-legal issues:

- putting patients interest first;
- communication;
- consent;
- confidentiality;
- complaints;

○ teamwork;
○ core professional development.
Other clinical governance issues:
- record keeping;
- child and vulnerable adult protection;
- prevention;
- staff training and involvement;
- clinical effectiveness;
- patient information and involvement;
- quality assurance and self-assessment (audit, peer review).

How would you handle this scenario?

Putting the patient's best interest first is the biggest factor here. Your first duty is to the patient, not the family. Keeping the patient's records confidential if he has capacity to consent is vital. The results will be confidential to the patient and must be discussed only with him unless he gives his permission for the information to be disclosed to the family.

Protecting elderly relatives is a natural response to potentially bad news. However, the patient's interests are best served by the protection of his information.

Protecting elderly patients is akin to protecting vulnerable adults and, in any case, no health professionals should break their oath by releasing patient information. The only circumstances are if information proves harmful to society or the patient. In these cases a court order needs to be presented.

This scenario needs to be treated delicately. Involvement of the wider dental team is advised and all staff should have appropriate training in handling breaking bad news.

The patient's family needs to be educated in the policy on confidentiality and it should be explained that results will be given to the patient first unless otherwise stated.

Your duty of care lies with the patient and records of any conversations, letters or demands need to be thoroughly documented in the notes to protect from any dento-legalities.

What are the future implications for managing risk?

Quality assurance needs to be reassessed. All CQC outcomes should have policies within the practice. All staff should have appropriate training when it comes to confidentiality, breaking bad news and communication, including complaints handling

There should be risk assessment of the practice to ensure appropriate information storage – locked cupboards, electronic backups, hard drives. All staff should have proper training in confidentiality and communication and in keeping CPD relevant, ensuring that all notes were adequate and that documentation included all conversations with the patient's family.

There should also be self-assessment – audit, peer review, reaudit, comparison to other clinicians, and reflection. Patient feedback will always aid in future communication.

GDC Standard: 5. Have a clear and effective complaints procedure

Scenario: A patient wants to complain with regards to how she was treated at the reception desk. She feels that the practice has failed, on numerous occasions, to meet her expectations. She asks you to direct her to the practice complaints procedure. You look in the policy folder and see that there is no complaints procedure document and a lot of the policies are out of date.

What are the clinical governance issues here?

How would you handle this scenario?

What are the future implications for managing risk?

What are the clinical governance issues here?

Dento-legal issues:
- putting patients' interests first;
- communication;
- consent;
- complaints;
- teamwork;
- core professional development;
- raising concerns.

Other clinical governance issues:
- record keeping;
- evidence-based practice;
- staff training and involvement;
- clinical effectiveness;
- patient information and involvement;
- quality assurance and self-assessment (audit, peer review).

How would you handle this scenario?

Immediately reassure the patient. Explain that you will take her details and send a copy as soon as possible. Try to resolve any matters there and then. Involve the wider team – the practice manager, the practice principal, your educational supervisor.

After the event, get a complaints procedure set up! The GDC clearly states that all practices must have 'a clear and effective complaints procedure'. A CQC inspection is also likely to want to see documentation of the practice complaints procedure when carrying out a practice inspection. In this case, the person to approach will be the practice manager, who has the responsibility to ensure that current policies on all governance aspects of the practice are documented. Explain to the patient that you will look into supplying the complaints procedure to her as soon as possible as it is currently being updated.

The complaints procedure should:
- be somewhere patients can view it easily;
- be easy to use;
- allow for quick resolutions;
- allow full and fair investigation;
- explain outcomes to patients clearly;
- improve service.

All members of the team must be appropriately trained. The complaints procedure is:
- to acknowledge receipt of the complaint as soon as you receive it by a phone call or in writing;
- contact your indemnity provider;
- there should be an acknowledgement within 3 working days;
- every 10 working days patients should be kept informed of progress with timescales.

The outcome should be:
- the result of fair investigation;
- an apology should be given;
- a solution should be provided for the complaint;
- solutions should be practical.

If patients are still not satisfied, they can contact NHS complaints or the Dental Complaints Service (private patients).

What are the future implications for managing risk?

All members of the team should learn from the complaint. There should be a practice meeting at which the complaint should be analysed. There should be CPD in complaint handling. Create a simple complaints procedure – all staff should be retrained in the procedure. There should be an audit and peer review.

GDC Standard: 6. Work with colleagues in a way that is in patients' best interests

Scenario: It is 4.30 p.m. on a Friday and an emergency patient has arrived wanting to be seen. You are the only dentist in the practice as most have gone home. The reception staff and nurses all want to go home and ask you to send the patient to NHS 111. Your closing times clearly state 5.30 p.m.

What are the clinical governance issues here?
What would you do on the day?
What would you do the day after?

What are the clinical governance issues here?

Dento-legal issues:
- putting patients' interests first;
- communication;

- complaints;
- teamwork;
- core professional development;
- raising concerns;
- personal behaviour control.

Other clinical governance issues:

- health and safety;
- record keeping;
- evidence-based practice;
- prevention;
- staff training and involvement;
- clinical effectiveness;
- patient information and involvement;
- accessibility;
- quality assurance and self-assessment (audit, peer review).

What would you do on the day?

You have a professional obligation to your patients until 5.30 p.m. This patient has rightly sought treatment within the hours in which you have offered your services. It would be legally and ethically wrong to close your doors to this patient.

It is unprofessional to send patients away if they are in pain. The GDC guidelines clearly state that all practitioners should not work alone so you need the support of the wider team. If the practice is open until 5.30 p.m. then the team is expected to stay until closing hours.

As the leader of the team in this scenario you should speak to the team to ensure that all parties – including reception and nurses – are on board with the plan. Sometimes you need to spend a little bit of extra time to ensure that patients are cared for and in this way the goodwill of the practice will increase. Emergency treatment does not often require a long time to complete and the wider team needs to understand that this is in the patient's best interest.

After seeing the patient and dealing with the pain, thank the team.

What would you do the day after?

Raise this issue with the wider team, practice manager, practice principal or a senior staff member – suggest a staff meeting to highlight the issues that arose. Arrange a team-building activity – if the team works well and clinically effectively together it enables a better running practice and better care for patients. Suggest CPD in patient care and management for all staff members. Suggest CPD in use of NHS 111 or other out-of-hours' services for all staff members.

Ensure the practice principal is aware about how staff feel about Friday afternoons and put a policy in place that everyone can look to when placed in difficult situations.

Audit time keeping – especially for Fridays. Peer review the issues raised.

GDC Standard: 7. Maintain, develop and work within your professional knowledge and skills

Scenario: You are 6 months into your DF1 training year. You notice that all of the radiographs that you take are too light and interpretation of radiographs all year has been challenging. All your radiographs are grade 2 or 3 quality. You find that no other dentist in the practice is justifying or grading radiographs and that for various reasons very few fall into grade 1 category. You have not realized the challenge you have been faced with until now and find it too embarrassing to say anything so far into your training year, especially if none of the other dentists have mentioned it. The films are developed in an automatic daylight developer, which looks quite old.

What are the clinical governance issues?

What are your general concerns?

What would you do to take this matter forward?

What are the clinical governance issues?

Dento-legal issues:

- putting patients' interests first;
- communication;
- complaints;
- teamwork;
- core professional development;
- raising concerns.

Other clinical governance issues:

- radiography;
- health and safety;
- record keeping;
- evidence-based practice;
- prevention;
- staff training and involvement;
- clinical effectiveness;
- quality assurance and self-assessment (audit, peer review).

What are your general concerns and what would you do to take this matter forward?

The taking of radiographs at this practice does not follow the recommended guidelines as set by the Ionising Radiation (Medical Exposure) Regulations 2000. Grade 2 radiographs are radiographs with minor errors that can still be diagnostically useful. However, high percentages of grade 2 in a practice must be investigated.

Having identified a problem that affects the whole practice, you need to take a team approach to resolve the issues. Approach the practice manager (neutral person) and find out whether a practice radiation protection officer has been appointed. Discuss your findings and suggest a practice meeting at which you discuss implementing an audit for the whole practice using the FGDP Standards in Dental Radiography as the set gold standard. The aim should be to identify how the practice is performing against the set standard and to then implement improvement. It is important to reaudit after the recommended time period to confirm that the practice standards have improved, thereby completing the audit cycle. Try to encourage the use of digital radiography and also encourage team members to attend CPD courses on the subject.

By implementing the above, you will be maintaining patient safety, demonstrating best practice and improving the standard of care. By involving the whole team you minimize the risk of blaming individuals and increase the awareness of the problem to the whole practice.

Remember that patients have the right to access their records at any point and if radiographs have not been justified or graded appropriately this shows a lack of training from staff and clinically effectiveness. The quality assurance of the practice will be raised and patients will feel unsafe within the practice. This could lead to complaints, which would not be in the best interest of the practice or best interest for the safety of patients.

GDC Standard: 8. Raise concerns if patients are at risk

Scenario: You have been working at a practice for some time and have been given an associate's diary to manage whilst he is away for a few weeks. You notice that a large proportion of his patients have undiagnosed periodontal disease and carious lesions. The patients do not seem to have been made aware of these findings. The majority of patients have not had a BPE and have a high percentage of bleeding on probing.

What are the clinical governance issues?

How would you manage this scenario?

What are the clinical governance issues?

Dento-legal issues:

- putting patients' interests first;
- communication;
- consent;
- confidentiality;
- complaints;

- ◦ teamwork;
- ◦ core professional development;
- ◦ raising concerns.

Other clinical governance issues:

- ◦ radiography;
- ◦ record keeping;
- ◦ evidence-based practice;
- ◦ prevention;
- ◦ staff training and involvement;
- ◦ clinical effectiveness;
- ◦ patient information and involvement;
- ◦ quality assurance and self-assessment (audit, peer review).

How would you manage this scenario?

This is an underperformance and a patient-care issue that needs to be addressed by the whole team rather than by blaming a named colleague. It is important to discuss your findings with the practice manager and a team meeting should be set up where the issues can be discussed in full. Make sure, after your appointment, to make contemporaneous notes in full with records of the witness (nurse) and justify your findings.

In order to ensure best practice throughout the team, an audit should be conducted that should include all dental associates and DCPs involved in periodontal care of patients. A small sample of patient records from each colleague should be taken and checked for the recording of BPE and subsequent treatment actions. The results should be compared against the chosen gold standard. This also gives you the optimum data with regard to the dentist in question.

A plan should then be implemented to improve the way periodontal disease is diagnosed and treated throughout the whole practice. Reauditing should be carried out after an appropriate time to see if improvement has been made.

Continuous professional development needs to be updated for all staff members, especially in periodontal disease, caries and delivering better oral health (DBOH).

Staff involvement and training internally needs to be managed – especially if staff need to raise a concern in the future.

By addressing the issue in this way, the whole practice benefits, the underperforming colleague is made aware of the changes that need to be made and everyone benefits.

Addressing the issue directly with the colleague could be counterproductive and should be discouraged, as that person will feel marginalized. This is about teamwork, not about blaming individuals. If, of course, this issue is across all patients the associate sees and the issue is far greater than suggested then a formal issue needs to be raised with the GDC.

GDC Standard: 9. Make sure your personal behaviour maintains patients' confidence in you and the dental profession

Scenario: A mutual dentist friend has uploaded a video from an alcohol-fuelled evening midweek, which you attended. The video does not look professional. The tag line states 'drunken dentist dancing'.

What are the clinical governance issues?

What will be your short-term management?

What will be your long-term management?

What are the clinical governance issues?

Dento-legal issues:

- putting patients' interest first;
- communication;
- consent;
- confidentiality;
- complaints;
- raising concerns;
- personal behaviour control.

Other clinical governance issues:

- health and safety;
- evidence-based practice;
- staff training and involvement;
- clinical effectiveness;
- patient information and involvement;
- quality assurance and self-assessment (audit, peer review).

What will be your short-term management?

Immediately ask for the photographs and tag line to be deleted. Speak to your indemnity provider about whether any actions need to be taken. Deal with any patient complaints. Speak to your educational supervisor in regards to advice.

What will be your long term management?

- Have a really good think about your actions – consider a log book or reflecting upon your actions.
- Speak to senior colleagues for advice.
- Do not let your personal behaviour reflect poorly on your professional standards.
- Set rules for yourself – including when you go out and have drinks. Stick to those guidelines to ensure you protect yourself and patients.

Patient communication scenarios

Communication scenarios are from the GDC, used with permission. Information is correct at the time of going to press. Please visit the GDC web site to check for any changes since publication: www.gdc-uk.org (accessed 10 November 2015).

Try these communication scenarios with a partner to practice how you deliver information.

You can split issues into dento-legal issues or clinical governance. See the lists below to help you talk through issues that may arise in the following scenarios:
Dento-legal issues:
- putting patients' interests first;
- communication;
- consent;
- confidentiality;
- complaints;
- teamwork;
- core professional development;
- raising concerns;
- personal behaviour control;
- patient information and involvement.

Clinical governance issues:
- infection control;
- radiography;
- health and safety;
- record keeping;
- child and vulnerable adult protection;
- evidence-based practice;
- prevention;
- staff training and involvement;
- clinical effectiveness;
- patient information and involvement;
- accessibility;
- quality assurance and self-assessment (audit, peer review).

1. Put patients' interests first
You are seeing a teenage girl for a routine examination. On investigation the palatal surfaces of her teeth have tooth wear. The history shows no aetiology of erosion from acidic drinks or foods; the patient is not pregnant or suffering from gastric problems. During the consultation the patient becomes very teary explaining she is suffering from bulimia. She is adamant that no one should find out and has asked you to keep this a secret.

2. Communicate effectively with patients

Explain periodontal disease and its managements to a patient with 433/4*34* BPE, bleeding on probing, a large amount of plaque and calculus stagnation. Radiographs show up to 60% bone loss with furcation involvement in the lower quadrants.

3. Obtain valid consent

A 12-year-old child attends with her 18-year-old stepsister holding a front tooth in her hand. It was knocked out 10 minutes ago in the park across the street. She seems otherwise unharmed but wants you desperately to help her.

4. Maintain and protect patients' information

An angry-sounding woman calls the practice, exclaiming that her husband has not returned home and asking the practice to give her the time he left his dental appointment today. You look in the diary and cannot see any appointment for the patient.

5. Have a clear and effective complaints procedure

A patient has attended today to speak to you and your practice manager regarding a complaint he has made against you and the practice. The patient had an extraction last week where the tooth broke and root was left *in situ*. When giving postoperative instructions you stated that the retained root should be left due to its proximity to the antrum and, if needs be, further surgery can be performed at a later date to have it removed. The patient claims that he was unaware of this complication.

6. Work with colleagues in a way that is in patients' best interests

A longstanding patient on bisphosphonates attends with emergency pain from a LL6. The patient had taken allendronic acid for 8 years and now is taking IV bisphosphonates. Radiographic evidence shows a large periapical radiolucency and clinically a mesio-occlusal carious lesion. It is your duty to communicate all options with the patient, including the wider team and specialists in this field.

7. Maintain, develop and work within your professional knowledge and skills

You see a 29-year-old girl for a new patient examination. Her primary complaint is her missing 'front tooth' and 'wonky smile'. On examination you see she has a class 1 molar relationship but her anteriors are in cross bite and she has a missing lateral incisor. The patient wants to work on television and wants a nice smile to give her some confidence. Discuss all options with the patient and explain that this treatment is out of your remit as it includes orthodontics and potential implant treatment. Patients may not always understand why one clinician cannot do all treatment. Try to explain the referral pathway to the patient and the different types of specialities.

8. Raise concerns if patients are at risk

You smell alcohol on an associate's breath as he walks into his surgery for his afternoon of patients. The next patient is about to be called in. You see he is very unsteady and fumbling over his clinical dental tray, trying to pick up instruments. He is in no way fit to treat patients. You need to have a conversation with him to persuade him not to treat patients this afternoon and to stop him from hurting himself and patients.

9. Make sure your personal behaviour maintains patients' confidence in you and the dental profession

You are seeing a 45-year-old male patient for a new patient full examination. You have done your examination and investigations and have taken relevant radiographs. It is evident that the patient suffers from moderate chronic periodontitis. His BPEs are 333/333. Radiographs show significant bone loss, especially in the molar region. The patient's risk factors include smoking and diabetes. You begin to explain the disease to the patient and highlight his risk factors, concentrating on smoking cessation. The patient exclaims how hypocritical this is considering he saw you a few weeks ago smoking at a local pub.

CHAPTER 7

Situational judgement test practice questions

CHAPTER MENU

Introduction

This section hosts 150 SJT questions – 75 of which are ranking based and 75 of which are best of three. Be reminded of the different type of SJT and how to determine your answer.

Section A: ranking-based SJTs

Candidates will be given a question with five possible responses to the specific situation in which they will then need to rank the five options from the most to least appropriate, usually from A to E.

Section B: 'best-of-three' based SJTs

The candidate will be presented with a situation question in which there will be eight possible answers. The candidate will then need to choose the **three most appropriate answers when considered together.**

The Dental Foundation Interview Guide: with Situational Judgement Tests, First Edition.
Zahid Siddique, Shivana Anand and Helena Lewis-Greene.
© 2017 John Wiley & Sons, Ltd. Published 2017 by John Wiley & Sons, Ltd.

Ranking-based SJTs: Questions

Questions are from the General Dental Council, used with permission. Information is correct at the time of going to press. Please visit the GDC web site to check for any changes since publication: www.gdc-uk.org (accessed 10 November 2015).

1 You overhear your receptionist telling a patient that the dentist looking after her is not very good and lazy. This is not the first time you have heard the receptionist speaking negatively about the clinical staff in the practice. The conversation between the patient and the receptionist has now moved on.

   Rank in order the following actions in response to this situation (A = most appropriate; E = least appropriate).

   a) Ignore what you heard and carry on with your day as normal.
   b) Immediately interrupt the receptionist and tell her she is being inappropriate in front of the patient.
   c) Wait till the end of the day and ask the receptionist to explain her comments.
   d) Report the receptionist to the practice manager.
   e) Inform your educational supervisor and ask for his advice on what to do.

2 Your educational supervisor asks you to work every Saturday, as he is currently short on staff with his regular Saturday dentist leaving for maternity leave. There are no other dentists in the practice available to work. You are already working Monday to Friday (9 a.m.–5 p.m.) and are finding the working week quite demanding.

   Rank in order the following actions in response to this situation (A = most appropriate; E = least appropriate).

   a) Report your educational supervisor to the GDC as you feel he is exploiting your contract hours.
   b) Politely say no as you feel this is against your contract hours.
   c) Agree because it will enhance your clinical experience.
   d) Ask your scheme leader for advice.
   e) Agree to carry out some Saturday shifts as long as the educational supervisor can arrange a regular day of in the week until he can find locum cover for Saturdays.

3 You refer Mr Patel, an 85-year-old patient, to the local oral medicine department after noticing a suspect lesion in the floor of the mouth during a routine examination. Later in the day you receive a call from Mr Patel's daughter asking you the reason why you have referred her dad to the oral medicine clinic.

   Rank in order the following actions in response to this situation (A = most appropriate; E = least appropriate).

   a) Explain to Mr Patel's daughter what you saw during her father's routine dental examination, making sure your explanations are without jargon, ensuring she understands what you are saying.

b) Tell the daughter that her father knows the reason and she will need to ask him.

c) Tell the daughter you suspect her father has a malignant lesion and have referred him for a second opinion.

d) Politely explain to the daughter that you are unable to talk to her about her father's care without his permission.

e) Tell the daughter that you are more than happy to discuss the referral further with her and her father at a new appointment as long as Mr Patel was happy for her to be there.

4 Your nurse asks you to see a patient in the waiting room, as he is looking pale and agitated. You are just about to see your next patient and are already running late on your appointments.

Rank in order the following actions in response to this situation (A = most appropriate; E = least appropriate).

a) You ignore the nurse and continue on with seeing your next patient, as you don't want to be more late with your appointments.

b) You ask your nurse to take your patient into the surgery and remain to attend to the patient in the waiting room.

c) Ask your nurse to call for another colleague to assist you.

d) Ask the receptionist to call for an ambulance for the patient in the waiting room.

e) You ask your nurse to invite the agitated patient in to your surgery and ask the receptionist to inform your next patient that you will be running 'a little late'.

5 You are very upset and angry after your DFT educational supervisor was rude and undermined you in front of a patient. This is not the first time he has done this and you feel he constantly undermines your clinical work.

Rank in order the following actions in response to this situation (A = most appropriate; E = least appropriate).

a) Speak to your DF1 educational supervisor at an appropriate time about the way you are feeling.

b) Discuss your educational supervisor's actions with your receptionist.

c) Behave as normally as you can so your educational supervisor does not see how angry and upset you are.

d) Reflect on whether you can learn from the feedback.

e) Tell your scheme leader how you are feeling, asking for advice on what you should do next.

6 You have arranged to go out to your best friend's birthday dinner tonight, which was planned a week ago. During lunch, your practice manager informs you that the mandatory practice meeting that was meant to take place

tomorrow morning has now been brought forward to tonight at the end of the working day.

Rank in order the following actions in response to this situation (A = most appropriate; E = least appropriate).

a) Pretend you forgot and leave as normal at the end of the day without anyone noticing.

b) Tell your nurse to inform the practice manager at the meeting that you couldn't make it.

c) Find out what the meeting is about and discuss with the person running the meeting whether your attendance is strictly necessary. Attend if required.

d) Call your friend and inform him that you cannot make the dinner as you have to stay in to work late.

e) Inform the person running the meeting that you can come in another day to catch up on the meeting notes and information if this is acceptable, as you would really like to attend your friend's birthday.

7 Your nurse, with whom you have had a good working relationship for the past 3 months, is beginning to arrive late for his shifts constantly, going from being 10 minutes late to now at times arriving half an hour late and not really giving you a suitable explanation. You managed to cover him on a few occasions by delaying your morning patients but it is now beginning to affect your work. He has also recently pressured you to finish early at the end of the day and not book long treatments after 4 p.m.

Rank in order the following actions in response to this situation (A = most appropriate; E = least appropriate).

a) Tell your educational supervisor and practice manger, asking for their advice about dealing with your nurse's timekeeping.

b) Discuss the problem with the other associate dentists in the practice to see if they've had a similar problem when they have worked alongside this nurse.

c) Speak to your nurse, asking him if there is a reason for his lateness and if there is anything you can do to aid him to arrive to work on time.

d) Speak to your nurse and tell him that his lateness is beginning to affect your clinical work and that you are no longer willing to delay your morning appointments as it is not in the best interest of the patient. Tell him he must be on time from now on otherwise you will make an official complaint about him to the principal dentist.

e) Make a record of each time he is late, then, at the end of the month, report him to the GDC.

8 You are in your second month of your DF1 job and are struggling to meet all your appointments as they have doubled from 10 patients per day in the first month to 20 patients per day in your second month. You find you are constantly against time and rushing through appointments. You are becoming increasingly anxious and stressed you may make a mistake. Your other DF1

colleagues seem to be getting on fine with seeing 20 patients per day and you feel you must be doing something wrong.

Rank in order the following actions in response to this situation (A = most appropriate; E = least appropriate).

a) Remain quiet about how you feel and hope things become easier for you to manage.

b) Speak to your educational supervisor, ask him for advice on patient-time management and make a strategic personal development plan with him where you gradually learn to work at a faster pace and feel safe and confident to do so at the same time.

c) Tell your educational supervisor you are not willing to see 20 patients per day and want to go back to only seeing 10 patients as you found this easier and safer to manage.

d) Ask your Df1 colleagues for tips on how they have managed to see an increased number of patients per day.

e) Tell the reception staff never to book more than 10–12 patients per day for you regardless of how busy the practice is.

9 Your nurse is becoming increasingly agitated with you, as you never finish on time. She has complained to you before that she does not like staying on late, as she does not get paid after 5 p.m. when her daily shift ends. You are trying your best to finish on time but find you are constantly being booked in with patients who require long difficult treatment as your late afternoon appointments.

Rank in order the following actions in response to this situation (A = most appropriate; E = least appropriate).

a) Tell the nurse she has no choice and needs to stay on late. She is not being a team player – remind her that you are not being paid for staying on late either.

b) Ask your educational supervisor for advice on effective patient time management.

c) Speak to your reception staff and ask them politely to make sure any appointments after 4 p.m. are routine checkups only.

d) Ask your practice manager to speak to the nurse.

e) Tell your nurse she can leave at 5 p.m. and continue to treat patients alone without her assistance.

10 You are on your weekly study day with the rest of your DF1 colleagues. During lunch, one of your close colleagues confides in you that he regularly smokes cannabis and has done so for the past few years. He has told you in confidence and is expecting you to support him.

Rank in order the following actions in response to this situation (A = most appropriate; E = least appropriate).

a) Review his clinical skills and performance on your study days. Report him to your training programme director (TPD) only if you are concerned about his performance.
b) Reassure your colleague that you will support him but urge him to speak to someone senior about his addiction as he is harming himself and could harm his patients. Warn him if he doesn't you will have no choice but to report him to his educational supervisor.
c) Report the matter to your colleague's DF1 educational supervisor.
d) Call your indemnity provider for advice.
e) Do not take the matter further and just hope your colleague resolves his addiction himself.

11 During your lunch break your nurse asks you if you can prescribe some antibiotics for her husband, as he has been experiencing toothache last 2 days, which is getting worse. She says he has a swelling coming from the gum and thinks it's a root infection. She informs you he is in a lot of pain and woke up with a fever today. He has not got a dentist and is very busy with work at the moment so hasn't got the time to see someone.

Rank in order the following actions in response to this situation (A = most appropriate; E = least appropriate).
a) Having checked with your nurse about her husband's medical history you prescribe metronidazole 200 mg and amoxicillin 250 mg and tell your nurse you are more than happy to see him when he does have time to come in for an appointment.
b) Tell your nurse not to diagnose her husband as it is out of her scope of practice.
c) Tell your nurse politely you do not want to prescribe antibiotics unnecessarily and that you don't mind seeing her husband in the practice at a time that suits him and then prescribe a suitable course of treatment if needed.
d) Tell your nurse you are not comfortable doing this and that she should ask another dentist in the practice.
e) Tell the nurse remote prescribing is not normal practice.

12 You have come back from lunch and realized your prescription pad is missing. The last time you remember using it is for a patient in the morning. It is normally kept locked in a draw in your surgery. The prescriptions are stamped by reception before patients leave the practice. The only people who have access are your nurse and the rest of the dental team.

Rank in order the following actions in response to this situation (A = most appropriate; E = least appropriate).
a) Immediately inform your educational supervisor.
b) Pretend that you have not realized and just continue with the rest of your day, opening a new prescription pad when needed.
c) Call your indemnity provider for advice.
d) Suspect your nurse has taken it and question her about it.
e) Call and notify the local clinical commissioning group (CCG).

13 Your DF1 educational supervisor has not been giving you regular tutorials. You speak to your DF1 colleagues on your study day and feel you are falling behind on the tutorial curricula and are at a disadvantage. Each time you have spoken to your educational supervisor regarding fitting tutorials in your calendar week, he has brushed you off. Recently he has said 'we will fit them in next week we still have plenty of time throughout the year.'

Rank in order the following actions in response to this situation (A = most appropriate; E = least appropriate).

a) Make a complaint about your educational supervisor to your patch associate dean.

b) Trust your educational supervisor's judgment and hope he does start to carry out some tutorials.

c) Speak to an associate in the practice who was previously a DF1 trainee in the practice and see if he can do some tutorials with you.

d) Approach your DF1 educational supervisor making a timetable for him scheduling in times for tutorials in accordance to his diary. Inform him you are deeply concerned that you are falling behind.

e) Report your educational supervisor to the GDC.

14 You have come in to work and noticed you have a patient in the afternoon who requires a difficult post-and-crown procedure on an upper right 7. Your educational supervisor is not in today and you have not carried out this type of treatment before and don't feel confident doing it without some supervision from your educational supervisor.

Rank in order the following actions in response to this situation (A = most appropriate; E = least appropriate).

a) Ask your reception staff to cancel the patient's appointment and to rebook on a date when your educational supervisor is working.

b) Continue as normal and hope the procedure goes smoothly.

c) Ask another dentist working in the practice to help you, going through the procedure with him before the appointment.

d) Have a look at the patient's treatment plan and carry out other treatment the patient requires, which you are more confident with. Reschedule the post and crown treatment at a later date when your educational supervisor will be in.

e) Ask another dentist working in the practice to see if he can treat the patient instead.

15 You find, after a month in to your DF1 year, that your DF1 educational supervisor is beginning to work less frequently with you in your practice. He has recently bought a new practice and is spending up to 4 days a week there. Last week he only came in for a few hours to check on your progress and left. You are concerned you are not getting the right amount of supervision and find it difficult to ask the other two part-time associates in the practice who are always very busy and are reluctant to help you when you require assistance or advice regarding a patient.

Rank in order the following actions in response to this situation (A = most appropriate; E = least appropriate).

a) Continue working as normal and hope that your educational supervisor will start spending more time at your practice when things settle down with his new practice.

b) Complain to your educational supervisor that he is not supporting you enough. Remind him he is not fulfilling his agreed educational supervisor contractual hours.

c) Make a complaint about your educational supervisor to your scheme leader without notifying your educational supervisor.

d) Ask the educational supervisor if he can speak to the associates to provide more support when he is not there.

e) Ask the practice manager for advice and to speak to your educational supervisor on your behalf.

16 You hear your nurse talking about your last patient to the practice manager in the staff room. The practice manager reveals the patient is the ex-husband of her best friend. The nurse goes on to say he had really bad teeth and had bad body odour. Your practice manager jokingly asks you 'if you had to double mask' and then continues asking you inappropriate questions about the appointment.

Rank in order the following actions in response to this situation (A = most appropriate; E = least appropriate).

a) Brush off the questions and pretend you need to leave the staff room straight away.

b) Not wanting to make it awkward or be rude, you join in the conversation adding a comment about the patient too – however, change the subject of the conversation quickly.

c) Immediately stop both of them and tell them they should not talk about patients in that way. Reminding them both the importance of patient confidentiality.

d) Report both to the principal dentist.

e) Before your next patient, politely speak to your nurse and remind her that she needs to respect patient confidentiality and never reveal details about a patient's appointment.

17 Your educational supervisor calls you at 8.30 in the morning on your day off asking if you can save the day and come in to work to cover the clinic of a colleague who has called in sick. The night before you were at your friend's birthday party and were out till the early hours and have woken up with a hangover. You feel you are not in the right state of mind to work as you consumed a large amount of alcohol the night before. What do you do?

Rank in order the following actions in response to this situation (A = most appropriate; E = least appropriate).

a) You agree to come in as soon as you can as you don't want to disappoint your educational supervisor.
b) You pretend you can't hear your educational supervisor on the phone and hang up, turning your phone off and going back to sleep.
c) You sympathetically inform your educational supervisor you have a full day planned ahead and are unable to come in.
d) You explain to your educational supervisor that you had a late night and don't feel you are in the right state of mind to work making it inappropriate for you came into work today.
e) You explain to your educational supervisor that you had a late night and therefore can only come in after lunch.

18 You are given an emergency patient towards the end of the day who is in some discomfort with toothache coming from his lower right posterior molar region. From his notes you can see the associate in the practice (the patient's regular dentist) has not taken any bitewings on this patient for the past 3 years, despite the patient having 6-monthly checkups. You feel strongly that if the patient had some bitewings taken at his last appointment his pain today could have been prevented. What are you going to do about this?

Rank in order the following actions in response to this situation (A = most appropriate; E = least appropriate).
a) Take the patient out of pain and refer back to the associate dentist.
b) Ask the patient if there is a reason as to why no bitewings were taken.
c) Take the patient out of pain. After the appointment, have a polite word with the associate regarding his patient and enquire as to why he did not take any bitewings for the patient.
d) Inform the principal dentist of the associate's actions after alleviating the patient from their pain.
e) Deal with the patient's emergency, take bitewings and inform the patient of your findings.

19 A 12-year-old patient attends with his elder brother (18 years of age) after sustaining a trauma injury at school resulting in subluxation of UR1. The patient is medically fit and well and has not sustained any head injuries. His older brother informs you both parents are abroad on holiday in Turkey.

Rank in order the following actions in response to this situation (A = most appropriate; E = least appropriate).
a) Refuse to treat the child especially as the mother is not present.
b) Reassure the patient and provide appropriate treatment for his trauma injury. Advise the patient and his brother to inform their parents about the injury and the treatment carried out as soon as possible.
c) Reassure the patient; provide the appropriate treatment for the patient's subluxation trauma on the UR1. Check the remaining dentition and stabilize the UR6 also as you notice a cavity present.

d) Call your educational supervisor into the surgery. Inform him you feel the child is Gillick competent and it is in the best interest of the patient to treat his trauma injury even though child's parents cannot be contacted presently.

e) Inform the patient and his brother to go to the local specialist paediatric dentist down the road who is more equipped to treat his injuries.

20 A nervous 25-year-old, fit-and-well female patient attends your surgery in pain. Your examination and radiographs reveal a diagnosis of acute reversible pulpitis on the UR7 that has an MO cavity. The patient is extremely needle phobic, anxious and worried the injection will hurt too much.

Rank in order the following actions in response to this situation (A = most appropriate; E = least appropriate).

a) Offer the patient a referral to a sedation specialist for treatment.

b) Use topical lidocaine and inject the anaesthetic as fast as possible.

c) Use topical lidocaine and inject the anaesthetic as slowly as possible.

d) Carry out treatment without a local anaesthetic.

e) Tell the patient she will have to put up with her anxiety; the pain from the local anaesthetic is less than what she is experiencing now.

21 You overhear the nurses discussing their CPD training certificates when one discloses to the other that majority of her training has been signed off from her father in law who is a retired dentist but she has not actually done the hours. She gives the other nurse his contact details and tells her to get in touch if she needs her CPD 'topping up'. What do you do?

Rank in order the following actions in response to this situation (A = most appropriate; E = least appropriate).

a) Ignore the situation as it is none of your business.

b) Speak to the practice manager showing your concerns and ask if she can intervene.

c) Report your nurses to the GDC anonymously.

d) Show your nurses the practice policy for CPD.

e) Bring up the issue at a practice meeting highlighting the nurses involved.

22 It is a Monday morning and all weekend it has been snowing heavily. It will almost be impossible to get to work on the icy roads but you do have a local bus stop nearby you could try; however, you know you will inevitably be late for your first patients.

Rank in order the following actions in response to this situation (A = most appropriate; E = least appropriate).

a) Call reception, explain the situation but still endeavour to go.

b) Pretend to be unwell and leave an answerphone message to cancel all your patients.

c) Message your practice manager to cancel your morning patients and say you will make it in for the afternoon.

d) Call your educational supervisor and explain the situation; seek his advice and act accordingly.

e) Don't go in – you know most patients will cancel anyway.

23 The practice has a Facebook account to share offers, promote the practice and deliver better oral health. You are browsing on the web page and can clearly see the Facebook account is commenting on other people's Facebook pages, clearly naming and shaming local dentists around the area. Whether this is an accident or not, whistleblowing is very serious and is taken seriously by the GDC. What do you do?

Rank in order the following actions in response to this situation (A = most appropriate; E = least appropriate).

a) Call a meeting highlighting the issue.

b) Make the practice manager aware of the comments so she can delete the contents.

c) Call your indemnity provider for confidential advice.

d) Keep a log book of events and record everything in your ePDP reflection.

e) Turn a blind eye for now but next time report this to the practice principal.

24 You have been a DF1 trainee for 3 weeks and at the end of a busy day your receptionist tells you that:

∘ Mrs Jones has returned saying that her socket has not stopped bleeding from the extraction this morning;

∘ Mr Smith has a huge swollen face and needs to be seen;

∘ Little Ronny who is 8 years old is with his mum with his front tooth in a jar of milk.

What do you do?

Rank in order the following actions in response to this situation (A = most appropriate; E = least appropriate).

a) Ask your senior colleague to see Ronny, tell your nurse to take Mrs Jones into your surgery where you place a pack into her mouth to stop the bleeding, then attend to Mr Smith.

b) Tell them that you are tired and that they should return tomorrow.

c) See little Ronny immediately as you know that the success of reimplantation is time dependent. Let the other patients wait.

d) Tell the receptionist to let patients know that they will all be seen and that you need the help of other colleagues.

e) Attend to Mr Smith as Ronny is not compliant and Mrs Jones has a thorough medical history, which you will need to talk through.

25 A very demanding patient wants you to 'cap' all her teeth as her friend had hers done in Europe and her smile looks fantastic now. The patient has anterior staining on her upper anterior with mild imbrication. There are no other clinical justifications for treatment. What do you do?

Rank in order the following actions in response to this situation (A = most appropriate; E = least appropriate).

a) Politely say no, explaining your rationale. Offer her alternative treatment for her staining and information regarding her imbrication.

b) Tell her you are referring her to specialist as you cannot do the treatment.

c) Call your educational supervisor in to help you deal with the situation.

d) Go ahead and do it as the patient wants the treatment and it would be good clinical experience for you.

e) Firmly say no, refusing to discuss it with her further and discharge from care.

26 You arrive on your first day as the new DF1. You look at your list and reception has booked a molar root-canal treatment for 45 minutes and a surgical extraction for 35 minutes. You know that this is an unrealistic expectation for you. What do you do?

Rank in order the following actions in response to this situation (A = most appropriate; E = least appropriate).

a) Say nothing as you do not wish to appear foolish and incapable on your first day.

b) Speak to your educational supervisor and see if the practice manager can try to adjust your books.

c) Ensure that reception are made aware of your capabilities and book accordingly.

d) Try and cope as best as you can – this is something that you need to get used to.

e) Ask your educational supervisor to assist you with the surgical and root-canal treatment to help you to carry out the work in the available time.

27 You are 20 minutes into a 30 minute appointment. It is 11.20 a.m. and your next patient, Mr Smith, is due at 11.30 a.m. You realize that treatment is going to take another 20 minutes to complete and you will be late seeing Mr Smith, who has yet has not arrived. What do you do?

Rank in order the following actions in response to this situation (A = most appropriate; E = least appropriate).

a) Continue as normal with your treatment as Mr Smith's timekeeping and attendance record is inconsistent.

b) Explain to the patient in the chair that the treatment will take longer than anticipated and apologize for the inconvenience this may cause.

c) Inform reception to tell Mr Smith you are running late. Tell the reception staff not to book any patients into your 'catch-up slots' to allow you to catch up with your notes and be on time for the rest of your appointments.

d) Rush through the treatment as you do not want to run late and are concerned you will not have enough time to write up all your notes.

e) Ask a colleague who is free if they can see Mr Smith when they arrive.

28 You have attended a party on Saturday night and have enjoyed yourself after a very stressful week in practice. You find out from a friend that photographs of you looking very drunk have appeared on Facebook. The person who has posted them has written that you are the local dentist and advises patients to cancel their appointments with you for the Monday morning. What do you do?

Rank in order the following actions in response to this situation (A = most appropriate; E = least appropriate).

a) Ask the person who posted the photographs to remove them as they do not realize the implications.

b) Threaten them that you will sue if they are not removed.

c) Ensure you are more careful regarding social media so this does not happen again in the future.

d) Seek help and advice from your indemnity provider.

e) In the event that a patient does complain (having seen the photographs) explain the circumstances and reassure the complainant that no patients were or are at risk as this was 2 days ago.

29 A new patient with poor oral hygiene and some cavities asks you to whiten their teeth. What would you do?

Rank in order the following actions in response to this situation (A = most appropriate; E = least appropriate).

a) Go ahead and sort the other stuff out later.

b) Explain the importance of a healthy mouth before you can commence the whitening.

c) Tell the patient that in your opinion they do not need their teeth whitened.

d) Give them an estimate for the whole treatment plan.

e) Refer them to your colleague down the road.

30 A new patient reveals that he is HIV positive to you. He is anxious that no one in his family knows. He asks you **not** to write it in the notes. What do you do?

Rank in order the following actions in response to this situation (A = most appropriate; E = least appropriate).

a) Eliminate all traces from his notes.

b) Lie to the patient and say you will not note it down but, after he leaves, update his medical history correctly.

c) Call your indemnity provider for advice.

d) Explain that the notes clearly need to reflect a full and contemporaneous medical history for his own safety but reassure him they will remain confidential.

e) Ask your educational supervisor to assist you with this patient's concern.

31 You are sitting in the pub opposite your practice where you observe three of the practice nurses laughing and joking about a patient that was seen today.

The patient could easily be identified from the conversation that you are over-hearing. What do you do?

Rank in order the following actions in response to this situation (A = most appropriate; E = least appropriate).

a) Ignore the situation as they should know better and you do not want to make a scene.

b) Speak to the person who is speaking the loudest privately so that he is aware of his inappropriate behaviour.

c) Challenge the whole group so that they are aware that their behaviour is inappropriate.

d) Tell the practice manager the next day.

e) Call your indemnity provider for advice.

32 You arrive early one morning and find your dental nurse scaling the teeth of a friend.

Rank in order the following actions in response to this situation (A = most appropriate; E = least appropriate).

a) Smile and say 'good morning' and go into the staff room to have your coffee as normal.

b) Realize that she should not be scaling teeth and speak with the practice manager.

c) Tell her to stop as it is outside her scope of practice and report the incident to the practice manager.

d) Call your indemnity provider.

e) Ask if she has done this before.

33 Social services suspect a 4-year-old patient is being neglected and want to know the details of her most recent attendances as well as your opinion on her dental health.

Rank in order the following actions in response to this situation (A = most appropriate; E = least appropriate).

a) Say nothing as you have an ethical duty to maintain patient confidentiality.

b) Release the information as it is in the patient's best interest.

c) Discuss it with your indemnity provider.

d) Discuss it with your educational supervisor/practice manager as soon as possible.

e) Do nothing.

34 Your colleague rushes into your surgery in a panic as he tells you that he has accidently cut his patient's lip with the bur. The patient is threatening to sue and has been left alone. What do you do?

Rank in order the following actions in response to this situation (A = most appropriate; E = least appropriate)

a) Reassure your colleague to return to the surgery and you will see that help is provided. It probably is not a good idea that the patient has been left alone.

b) Ask your nurse to stay with your patient while you attend to your colleague's patient.

c) Ask your nurse to stay with your patient and call the practice manager to attend to your colleague while you attend to his patient.

d) Tell your colleague to call their indemnity provider.

e) Carry on as though nothing had happened.

35 A 6-year-old child attends your clinic showing serious bruising on his neck and inner arm region. He is withdrawn and the mother seems uninterested in your clinical work but more concerned about the cost and prices.

Rank in order the following actions in response to this situation (A = most appropriate; E = least appropriate).

a) Speak to your educational supervisor and ask him to see the child for a second opinion.

b) Record your examination, take pictures and ask your nurse to log her opinions too.

c) Call your indemnity provider for information advice.

d) Call child social services for informal advice.

e) Reflect upon this on a scheme study day and ask peers for advice.

36 You are finding it difficult in the first few months as your educational supervisor has given you the task of training up one of the junior nurses. You are not finding anything clinically challenging; however, getting used to a new environment, the computer system and timekeeping plus training the nurse is difficult. What do you do?

Rank in order the following actions in response to this situation (A = most appropriate; E = least appropriate).

a) Keep a close eye on her as it does not matter whether you run behind.

b) Speak to your personal training programme director asking for advice on how to go about this.

c) Bring this up at a staff meeting insisting you want to change nurses.

d) Reflect upon this in your ePDP and see how it goes over the next few weeks.

e) Speak to your educational supervisor to reorganize how you are working at present.

37 You attend a CPD course on infection control within the practice. The instructions are that all healthcare professionals must wash their hands using the modified Ayliffe technique. Your nurse states that some of the associates do not use this technique and expresses her concerns on the matter. The practice principal seems dismissive of her comment and the meeting continues. You feel concerned about her comment. What do you do?

Rank in order the following actions in response to this situation (A = most appropriate; E = least appropriate).

a) Bring up the comment to the practice principal later on, asking for an investigation into this to take place.

b) Do a clinical audit to monitor the practice infection control and bring any findings up at the next practice meeting for a peer review.

c) Write a diary logging all infection control issues you have noted to be brought up at the next practice meeting.

d) Ask the other associates of their opinions on the nurses comments, if they agree then take this to the practice principal for further training.

e) Note the nurse's comment and always try to wash hands in between.

38 Six months into your DF1 year, you are starting to see a mixture of private and NHS patients. A few of the NHS patients are asking for treatments that are private but wanting to pay NHS prices. It is very easy to do so as all materials are kept in the same surgery and it would be great for your clinical portfolio; however, you know this is unethical and a violation of the NHS contract. One patient asks for a white filling for aesthetic reasons only where an amalgam filling is as suitable clinically. You know this is not NHS protocol but the patient keeps urging you to do so. What do you do?

Rank in order the following actions in response to this situation (A = most appropriate; E = least appropriate).

a) Explain the NHS versus private treatments issues to the patient and kindly suggest she pays privately if she prefers a white filling.

b) Explain your concerns to your educational supervisor as the line between treatments is becoming blurred and you need further guidance.

c) Ask the patient to see another dentist as you can only treat her under the NHS guidelines.

d) Treat the patient with a white filling as you feel it is as suitable and subsidize her cost to NHS pricing if she allows you to take photos for your portfolio.

e) Ask your TPD if you can be moved from this practice as the patients have extremely high expectations.

39 You are running late after a busy day. You had scheduled extra CPD training after work but will unfortunately be unable to attend. You call to cancel the training however a few days later receive an automated CPD certificate in an email. What do you do?

Rank in order the following actions in response to this situation (A = most appropriate; E = least appropriate).

a) Delete the email. It would be unethical to add the certificate to your CPD if you weren't in attendance.

b) Print the certificate out and add it to your CPD.

c) Reply to the CPD training course asking if you can add this to CPD even if you were not in attendance.

d) Inform the CPD training providers of the error and reschedule your CPD training to ensure you are not falling behind on your CPD hours.

e) Speak to your educational supervisor for further advice on this error.

40 Your educational supervisor approaches you at lunch and speaks to you about your current activity report. He points out that in the past 3 months you have carried out and completed lots of band 3 treatment and his lab bill is very high because of you. He asks you to do fewer crowns and says you should do large fillings instead and only do crowns and bridges if a patient is paying privately. This is not the first time he has bought up the issue of high lab bills and is now is expecting you to do less lab-based treatment.

Rank in order the following actions in response to this situation (A = most appropriate; E = least appropriate).

a) Accept your educational supervisor's wishes and don't plan for crowns or bridges for NHS patients, even when they are required.

b) Inform your educational supervisor you have only carried out crowns or bridges when they have been in the best interest of the patient and will continue practising in that manner.

c) Only offer crown and bridge treatments to your patients privately if clinically indicated or offer to refer them to another NHS dentist.

d) Ask your TPD for advice.

e) Report your educational supervisor to the GDC.

41 You are seeing a child for a routine examination at the start of your DF1 year. The child seems withdrawn, quiet and nervous and mother seems uninterested. You see a large bruise on the side of the patient's neck and bite marks in the inside of the lip. The child's mother steps outside to take a phone call when the child reveals to you their stepfather abuses them. You look back in the notes to see the previous dentist has not noted anything but the child's sombre attitude, which he put down anxiety about dentistry. What do you do?

Rank in order the following actions in response to this situation (A = most appropriate; E = least appropriate).

a) Write full contemporaneous notes documenting all you have seen from the examination, ask your nurse to do the same and call the family in for a review in a week.

b) Write full contemporaneous notes documenting all you have seen from the examination and inform the mother she needs to contact social services for the child's wellbeing.

c) Write full contemporaneous notes documenting all you have seen from the examination. Call your indemnity provider for advice.

d) Call your educational supervisor for a second opinion. State what you have found to the mother and inform her child services will be called immediately.

e) Ask your nurse to stay with the child. Speak to your educational supervisor and the safeguarding lead in your practice about your concern and call child services immediately to ensure the safety of your patient. Inform the mother.

42 You are late at work one evening and walk past the reception desk where you see that the head receptionist is taking cash from the desk and placing it into her bag. She sees you and panics, exclaiming that she just needs extra money for her son's lunch this week and she assures you that she will replace it, begging you not to tell anyone what you have seen. What do you do?

Rank in order the following actions in response to this situation (A = most appropriate; E = least appropriate).

a) Tell her to put the money back and report her actions to the practice manager.

b) Agree to not say anything as long as she replaces the money in due course.

c) Tell her to put the money back and report her actions to the principal dentist.

d) Bring up the importance of team work, respect for practice rules and the workers behaviour at a practice meeting.

e) Reassure your receptionist and tell her regardless of the situation she should put the money back as it is wrong to take cash from the desk without permission and that you will help her to speak with the practice manager together to arrange some support for her.

43 A patient you see for periodontal treatment does not want to disclose his medical history and asks what a quick clean has got to do with his medicines.

Rank in order the following actions in response to this situation (A = most appropriate; E = least appropriate).

a) Politely explain how medical history is of importance before carrying out any treatment.

b) Stop the appointment there and then refuse to treat the patient.

c) Continue with the treatment as realistically what are the chances of anything happening.

d) Explain the situation to your educational supervisor and ask him how he deals with such patients.

e) Speak to your TPD about the difficult patients you are experiencing on DF1 and ways to manage them.

44 You notice that your nurse does not dry flush the chair at the end of the day for 2 minutes as required. What do you do?

Rank in order the following actions in response to this situation (A = most appropriate; E = least appropriate).

a) Tell the practice manager your concerns.

b) Teach your nurse how to set up the dental chair, explaining the importance of dry flushing.
c) Ask the head nurse to suspend your nurse for her behaviour.
d) Draw up a clinical audit with your nurse on infection control in the practice.
e) Ask the practice principal for a new nurse who is more competent.

45 You are placing a bridge on a 70-year-old patient. The fit is good – not exceptional but it does the job; however, the colour is not correct and you have to adjust the bite significantly so you can now see the metal coping. You feel you could do a better job but you know it will cost the practice in lab fee bills. What do you do?

Rank in order the following actions in response to this situation (A = most appropriate; E = least appropriate).
a) Just fit the bridge – the patient is elderly and will not mind about aesthetics too much.
b) Explain all your concerns to the patient and, if the patient consents, fit the bridge.
c) Tell the patient you are not happy with the bridge and send it to the lab for a remake, charging the patient for the lab fee.
d) Personally subsidize the lab fee for the patient.
e) Call the laboratory and explain your clinical findings asking if they can come for a consultation to make the bridge together.

46 You are placing an omnimatrix band on a large first molar that is proving to be difficult. The matrix band keeps breaking after having a few attempts to fit in. You are struggling to get it to fit but do not want to ask for help on such a trivial matter. What do you do?

Rank in order the following actions in response to this situation (A = most appropriate; E = least appropriate).
a) Call your educational supervisor in to help assist with the matrix band, swallowing your pride.
b) Audit all your matrix-band placements.
c) Temporize the tooth and rebook the patient for a later date ensuring you have practiced matrix-band placements.
d) Ask an associate who is available to help you place the matrix band.
e) Avoid treating cavities requiring matrix bands.

47 You only have 2 days of annual leave left but really want to attend a sought-after 3-day dental course during your DF1 year. What do you do?

Rank in order the following actions in response to this situation (A = most appropriate; E = least appropriate).
a) Attend the course. Plan to call in sick at your practice so you can attend the third day.

b) Ask your educational supervisor for options in regards on what to do even if this may jeopardize your chances of going on the course.

c) Ask your TPD about what can be done in regards to this situation.

d) Try to find a 2-day course to attend instead, even if it is not as sought after.

e) Stop searching for courses and focus on the basics.

48 Your patient asks you what is wrong with your receptionist. He goes on to say she is always so miserable and abrupt when she communicates.

   Rank in order the following actions in response to this situation (A = most appropriate; E = least appropriate).

a) Laugh with the patient and ignore the comment.

b) Call the receptionist in straight away and ask her to apologize to the patient.

c) Apologize to the patient and reassure him that she is a valuable member of the team.

d) Inform your DF1 educational supervisor of the patient's comments, asking him to speak to the receptionist.

e) Speak to the receptionist when suitable and give her some polite advice and tips on how to improve her communication skills.

49 A patient comes in to see you complaining of pain from his lower premolar tooth. He describes the pain as having been intermittent for the past 2 months. It has grown progressively worse in the past 3 days and he now has a facial swelling. On completion of your examination and radiographs, you diagnose the patient with chronic periapical periodontitis. You inform the patient that he requires root-canal treatment to save the tooth and a course of antibiotics. The patient is happy to go ahead with the treatment but has asked you to write him a letter addressing his diagnosis so he can show his university, as he has missed some coursework deadlines in the past 2 days and needs to show them some evidence. Your best opinion is that the patient will require no more than 1 or 2 days' rest; however, the patient is insisting that you should write he requires at least 4 weeks rest as his body takes longer than usual to recover from bacterial infections.

   Rank in order the following actions in response to this situation (A = most appropriate; E = least appropriate).

a) Write 4 weeks' rest to avoid any further disagreement.

b) Compromise with the patient by writing 2 weeks' rest.

c) Ask your educational supervisor for advice in regards to the letter and to come in to help you explain circumstances to the patient.

d) Write that you recommend 1 week's rest and advise the patient to come back to see you or his GP if he is still feeling unwell.

e) Only write what you feel the patient's diagnosis and recovery time will be in the letter and explain to the patient that the combination of the root-canal treatment and antibiotics is usually sufficient in controlling the infection.

50 You are seeing a patient for whom you had treatment planned at the beginning of your DF1 year. He required endodontic treatment with the placement of a post. You have completed all the preventative treatment and the endodontic treatment. Today is the placement of the post. You are excited to do this as you have never done one before. You have spent your tutorial time preparing for the post and have read lots of journals to aid today's appointment. You see that you educational supervisor is not in today as she is unwell; however, one of the other associates is in but you have never discussed this case with him in the past. What do you do?

Rank in order the following actions in response to this situation (A = most appropriate; E = least appropriate).

a) Brief the associate on your case, seek his advice and proceed if applicable, knowing he is there to assist and aid if needed.

b) Call your educational supervisor at home and complain how he is not here to support you adequately.

c) Go ahead with the treatment as planned without asking anyone for help as you are familiar with the information you gathered from your tutorials and all the journals you read.

d) Cancel the patient's appointment and reschedule for a day when your educational supervisor is available.

e) See your patient but do not do the post placement and get on with other treatments, with which you are confident.

51 Your practice refers anything out of its remit of scope to a local specialist dental practice as well as a hospital. You start to notice a lot of the patients referred to the specialist practice for implants do not return to your practice. You ask the reception team to call these patients for their recalls with the majority replying that they now attend the specialist dental practice for all their treatment. You are appalled that this practice is stealing your patients. What do you do?

Rank in order the following actions in response to this situation (A = most appropriate; E = least appropriate).

a) Write up what you have found in a log diary with reception staff contributing too – bring this up at a staff meeting to decide what to do next as a team.

b) Call your indemnity provider for advice.

c) Change the specialist dental practice you refer to so this issue does not occur again.

d) Tell your educational supervisor and ask him to call a meeting with the specialist practice to discuss the patients that have been referred to them.

e) Call CQC and anonymously make a complaint about the specialist practice.

52 One of the associates openly tells you that he does not treat female patients due to his religious beliefs and therefore not to refer any to him. He is the only oral surgeon in the practice, so any complicated extractions or surgical procedures are usually referred to him.

Rank in order the following actions in response to this situation (A = most appropriate; E = least appropriate).

a) Refer patient to the oral surgeon and ignore what he has told you about his beliefs as under GDC guidelines he must treat all patients equally.

b) Bring up the referral issue with your educational supervisor, asking for his advice.

c) Refer patients to a local hospital unit even though the waiting list is longer.

d) Bring up the issue of him not treating woman with the raising concerns lead, asking him to raise this issue.

e) Read the GDC guidelines to the oral surgeon and tell him you will not comply with his request.

53 Mrs Jones, a new patient, requests that you replace her four upper anterior crowns. She has had them for 20 years and she is bothered by the black margins, which are visible. She has not seen a dentist for 10 years. She reports no symptoms. You take radiographs, which show large areas of secondary caries around the crown margins and up to 75% bone loss around some of the teeth. Two of the teeth have posts and apical radiolucencies.

Rank in order the following actions in response to this situation (A = most appropriate; E = least appropriate).

a) Explain your findings and provide all relevant treatment options.

b) Provide all crowns as this is the patient's primary concern.

c) Tell her that she will need all four teeth extracted and an immediate denture fitted.

d) Refer her to a restorative specialist for a second opinion.

e) Tell the patient there's little you can do to help and its best to monitor the teeth.

54 Mr S attends your surgery alone expecting an extraction. Your nurse tells you that he doesn't speak much English. He has a note to say that he is now on Warfarin. His wife speaks English but is at home.

Rank in order the following actions in response to this situation (A = most appropriate; E = least appropriate).

a) Take out the tooth as you have all the appropriate haemostatic agents that you need.

b) Call Mrs S and explain that you cannot carry out the treatment as you do not have a full medical history and there is a consent issue as he does not speak English. Ask if she can come in to translate and bring with her the necessary medical documents for a later appointment that day.

c) Arrange for a translator to attend the next visit if Mrs S cannot attend and rebook.

d) Ask one of the nurses who speaks the language to explain to Mr S why you cannot proceed.

e) Refer him to your in-house oral surgeon.

55 A woman calls reception at the practice and demands to know if her husband has attended and also wants details of his treatment. She sounds angry!

Rank in order the following actions in response to this situation (A = most appropriate; E = least appropriate).

a) Give her all the details as she sounded very angry.

b) Tell her that you will call her back after you discuss it with someone senior.

c) Call the man and inform him.

d) Tell her that this information is confidential and that if she wishes to find out she needs to talk directly with her husband.

e) Tell her he attended but don't provide any details regarding his treatment.

56 You and a fellow dental colleague are at a bar. It is getting late and you both have a long journey home. Both of you have an early clinic tomorrow. However, your friend does not want to leave.

Rank in order the following actions in response to this situation (A = most appropriate; E = least appropriate).

a) Wait with him and ensure you have enough caffeine to get you through the day tomorrow.

b) Try to persuade him to leave; remind him of the early clinic he has and his responsibility towards his patients.

c) Stay with him, enjoy your night and plan to call in sick tomorrow; that way no patients will come to harm.

d) Call his educational supervisor and practice tomorrow informing them of his behaviour last night.

e) Remind him of his early clinic and leave alone as you don't want to jeopardize your work tomorrow.

57 Your TPD advises you on your first study day that you are not to do private work as a priority but should concentrate mostly on the NHS aspect of dentistry. However, when you start your foundation dentist (FD) training you get the feeling your educational supervisor is pushing a lot of private work on you. What do you do?

Rank in order the following actions in response to this situation (A = most appropriate; E = least appropriate).

a) Speak to your TPD, seeking advice.

b) Negotiate a deal with your educational supervisor where you earn from private work to make it worth your while.

c) Do as you are told by your educational supervisor.

d) Tell your educational supervisor that you should be focusing on NHS treatments.

e) Tell your practice manager about how you are feeling overwhelmed with private work.

58 A school teacher arrives at reception with one of the schoolchildren as an emergency. She shows you the child's tooth (UR1), which is in a solution in a small pot. The teacher informs you the tooth avulsed 20 minutes ago. The tooth is not fractured.

Rank in order the following actions in response to this situation (A = most appropriate; E = least appropriate).
a) Reimplant the tooth immediately with no follow up.
b) Ask a senior associate to reimplant immediately.
c) Reimplant the tooth immediately. Arrange a follow-up appointment as soon as possible with the child's parents also attending.
d) Refer the child to the nearest ADC hospital department.
e) Rearrange the appointment as soon as possible, with valid consent.

59 Your practice is running low on nursing staff, with a few unwell. The head nurse has organized a locum nurse to attend the morning clinic. You will be working with the locum nurse today; however, before you go into the surgery another longstanding nurse quietly speaks to you stating that she can smell alcohol on the replacement nurse's breath.

Rank in order the following actions in response to this situation (A = most appropriate; E = least appropriate).
a) Speak with the locum nurse to assess if she has been drinking alcohol, if so, Inform her she will not be able to work as its not in the best interest of the patients.
b) Inform the locum agency of what has occurred and ask them to send you another nurse as soon as possible.
c) Bring the issue of shortness of staff and the incident up at the weekly team meeting to ensure such an incident does not occur again.
d) See patients as normal; you are low on nurses and you can manage anyway.
e) Call an emergency meeting with the other two dentists on site asking for their advice.

60 You are having regular tutorials with your educational supervisor and really enjoying the practical tutorials but when it comes to theoretical tutorials you realize that your tutor is teaching you material that is not evidence based and out-of-date
theory. You suspect he is unaware of new and current research.

Rank in order the following actions in response to this situation (A = most appropriate; E = least appropriate).
a) Speak to your TPD about your findings, seeking advice and keeping a log book of tutorials.

b) Write up your tutorials on the ePDP, highlighting the incorrect theory in the hope that your educational supervisor reads it.

c) Sign up your educational supervisor to extra CPD training days, hoping he will get the hint.

d) Speak to another associate dentist to give you theoretical tutorials instead.

e) Show your educational supervisor articles and journals with up-to-date information so you can discuss them with him.

61 You are seeing a new patient who asks if you can replace his sound silver fillings with white fillings on his posterior teeth under the NHS. He goes on to say that he will allow you to take photos of it for your portfolio and, as you are young, you will need this to promote your skills.

Rank in order the following actions in response to this situation (A = most appropriate; E = least appropriate).

a) It will be good for your portfolio so carry out the treatment under the NHS, giving clinical reasons to justify the treatments in the notes.

b) Ask the practice principal permission to treat the patient privately but charge him the same as he would pay under the NHS, giving your reason as the fact that it would be good experience for you.

c) Ask your educational supervisors for a second opinion on how to handle this scenario.

d) Tell the patient you cannot justify composite materials under the NHS; however, if this was done privately fees can be worked out accordingly.

e) Ask the patient to leave the practice for making such an unethical proposition.

62 You are midway extracting a lower right molar when the tooth breaks coronally and all you can see are the retained roots, which are embedded under the gingival level. This procedure will need surgical intervention. As an undergraduate you only completed one surgical extraction and it was under supervision.

Rank in order the following actions in response to this situation (A = most appropriate; E = least appropriate).

a) Continue with the procedure. You know the theory and it will be good for your experience.

b) Stop the procedure, calling in an experienced dentist to help.

c) Leave the retained root in and rebook the patient when your educational supervisor is available to supervise the surgical procedure.

d) Leave the root and place a suture on top, not informing the patient about what happened.

e) Persevere with hand instruments as eventually the tooth must come out.

63 Your nurse has been practising for 15 years and tells you she is not registered with the GDC.

Rank in order the following actions in response to this situation (A = most appropriate; E = least appropriate).

a) Explain the implications of her disclosure, encouraging her to register immediately.
b) Call your educational supervisor immediately and force the nurse to confess.
c) Speak to the practice principal immediately, explaining the situation.
d) Log the nurse's confession and watch her closely.
e) Dismiss her confession.

64 You are enjoying your FD year a lot. However when you attend study days you realize you are receiving more coursework from your educational supervisor than your peers do. You do like your educational supervisor as he is a nice man; however, now you feel overwhelmed with work, being made to do audits and practice policy writing. You feel you are doing the work of a practice manager alongside being an FD.

Rank in order the following actions in response to this situation (A = most appropriate; E = least appropriate).

a) Speak to your TPD showing him the list of extra work you have had to do and ask for advice.
b) Speak to your educational supervisor asking why you are being treated unfairly.
c) Speak to your educational supervisor asking why you have so much extra work to do and how all of it is relevant to your FD year.
d) You like your educational supervisor and want to keep good relations so continue doing the work for him.
e) Try and convince your educational supervisor of the need to hire a practice manager.

65 You have two educational supervisors. You have a very amicable relationship with one; however, the other patronizes you, undermines your clinical assessments and generally ignores you. You are finding it quite upsetting and dislike going to work.

Rank in order the following actions in response to this situation (A = most appropriate; E = least appropriate).

a) Speak to the other educational supervisor in confidence telling him how you are feeling and ask him to provide you with insight on why the other educational supervisor acts this way.
b) Speak to your TPD for advice on what can be done to improve your relationship.
c) Seek help from the other FDs in your scheme. They may be experiencing a similar issue.
d) Discuss the matter at a practice meeting.

e) Confront your educational supervisor when he undermines you in front of a patient for all to see.

66 You are seeing a patient for a routine extraction of a retained root. As you extract the root, the crown on the adjacent tooth falls off. What do you do?

Rank in order the following actions in response to this situation (A = most appropriate; E = least appropriate).

a) Inform the patient immediately of what has happened, reminding him that this was one of the possible risks discussed during consent.
b) Give the patient postoperative instructions, and ask him to come see you tomorrow to recement the crown.
c) Throw the crown away the patient will never know.
d) Speak to your nurse and tell her to mix cement quickly and recement whilst the patient is numb as she will not realize.
e) Call your educational supervisor to come and help you explain this bad news to the patient.

67 The ultrasonic handpiece has stopped working in your surgery. You notice your afternoon has several periodontal patients, all needing root surface debridement subgingivally. What do you do?

Rank in order the following actions in response to this situation (A = most appropriate; E = least appropriate).

a) Try to swap surgeries within the practice with one that has a working ultrasonic scaler.
b) Ask reception to cancel all afternoon appointments as you cannot work like this.
c) See all periodontal patients. Explain to them what has happened and do six-point pocket charts where applicable or any fillings needed instead. Rebook when handpiece has been repaired.
d) Use a hand scaler even though you know it will not give a good result. Explain to the patients that they will need to come back for further appointments when the handpiece has been repaired.
e) Use a slow handpiece and polish the patients teeth instead as they will not know the difference.

68 You have been sent your audit back a few times by the scheme assistant as it is not to an appropriate standard. You are unsure how to improve it and what to do in this instance. What do you do?

Rank in order the following actions in response to this situation (A = most appropriate; E = least appropriate).

a) Speak to your practice manager and ask to borrow the old DF1s audits to copy.
b) Speak to the assistant and ask for better feedback than just sending it back to you.

c) Take the audit to your educational supervisors and ask for a tutorial on how to improve.

d) Speak to the TPD, asking her why you are receiving the audit back so much.

e) Keep trying as you will get there in the end.

69 You have two educational supervisors who are split between two DF1s. You both call over one educational supervisor much more than the other for second opinions and feedback. The other educational supervisor is slow getting to you, he patronizes you in front of patients and tutorials are always cut short. This is not fair on the one educational supervisor as you can see the two of you are tiring him out. What can you do?

Rank in order the following actions in response to this situation (A = most appropriate; E = least appropriate).

a) Hold a meeting between your educational supervisors and trainees with a mediator to discuss the issues at hand.

b) Call your TPD, explaining how you feel, and gain an understanding of how to pursue this.

c) Do not worry about the complacent educational supervisor; it is his fault he acts this way.

d) Speak to your fellow DF1 and brainstorm what to do next together.

e) Tell all the associates to be on call if either of you need them as one educational supervisor is useless.

70 Your nurse drops a spatula on the floor, picks it up and continues to use it mixing alginate.

Rank in order the following actions in response to this situation (A = most appropriate; E = least appropriate).

a) Signal to her to start mixing again with a new spatula and speak to her and the head nurse after, as this is poor infection control.

b) Shout at her in front of the patient, asking her to rethink what she is doing.

c) Stop the procedure and ask for another nurse to attend your clinic.

d) Pretend you have not seen this poor infection control action and continue as you are running late.

e) Politely ask your nurse to remix using a new spatula and help her understand the consequences of her actions.

71 It is a Friday evening and you are writing up some notes, referral letters and generally checking all is in order for the following week. All the other associates have left the practice and the nurses are nearly finished tidying up. The receptionist enters your surgery demanding you to finish, as she needs 30 minutes to back up the system. She sits in your surgery watching you and constantly pressurizing you to hurry up. You are finding this very stressful and cannot check your notes properly.

Rank in order the following actions in response to this situation (A = most appropriate; E = least appropriate).

a) Politely ask the receptionist to leave your surgery as she is distracting you and notes will be finished quicker without her present.

b) Stop what you are doing there and then and shut down the computer – you most likely are done anyways.

c) Call your educational supervisor to return to the practice as the team is giving you a hard time.

d) Quickly rush through your notes and do not double check them.

e) Ask your nurse to help you diffuse the situation with the receptionist as you are under pressure.

72 You and your colleagues find your weekly study days are not very productive. Each week your TPD arrives late, doesn't reply to his emails and doesn't cover the topic of discussion very well. He is more interested in leaving the day early to go for drinks with the group. He is very sociable but you do not find him to be a good teacher.

Rank in order the following actions in response to this situation (A = most appropriate; E = least appropriate).

a) Express your concerns with your DF1 peers to the TPD as a collective group.

b) Seek advice from another TPD on a different scheme on what to do.

c) Report the TPD to the head of the deanery.

d) Ask your educational supervisors collectively to speak with the TPD.

e) Ignore his behaviour. Study days are meant to be more social and relaxed.

73 You are struggling with your health at work. You have a problem with your back and never told anyone on the deanery about your medical background. After the first month in your DF1 year, your back pain has grown much worse; it feels stiffer and the more patients you treat the worse the pain is becoming. You are feeling the stiffness in your back even when you are not working. You are trying your best to focus on your posture and not to arch your neck to much but find it too difficult to see using your mirror alone.

Rank in order the following actions in response to this situation (A = most appropriate; E = least appropriate).

a) Try to power through and hope that with experience your posture and use of the mirror will improve.

b) Ask your educational supervisor for tips and supervision on your posture and use of the mirror.

c) Ask your educational supervisor/practice manager for a few days off to rest your back, allowing it to heal.

d) Do not tell anyone – just call in sick as you know your health is important.

e) Ask your educational supervisor for a new chair, which may improve your posture.

74 Your nurse tells you after an appointment how bad at communicating you were. She says you need to speak slower, explain what you are doing methodically and if that was her she would not have felt reassured in your clinical assessment. What do you do?

Rank in order the following actions in response to this situation (A = most appropriate; E = least appropriate).

a) Ignore her as she is not your educational supervisor and cannot speak to you this way.

b) Tell the deanery that you want to change training practices as the team is rude to you.

c) Ask your nurse to attend your next tutorial and discuss with your educational supervisor how to improve.

d) Ask your nurse to write down advantages and disadvantages of your communication skills for you to reflect upon.

e) Ask your educational supervisor for a new nurse as you feel she has undermined and insulted you.

75 You have your end-of-year signoffs and realize there is a quota list with rough guidelines on what is needed to complete the year. You realize that you have done no bridges all year. What do you do?

Rank in order the following actions in response to this situation (A = most appropriate; E = least appropriate).

a) Tell your educational supervisor that you are low on bridges.

b) Tell your TPD that you are low on bridges and to have an extension.

c) Put through one bridge on your weekly log – no one will notice.

d) Ask your scheme peers what situation they are in and see whether they can advise and guide you on further steps to take.

e) Do nothing – it will be fine in the end.

Ranking-based SJTs: Answers

Answers are from the General Dental Council, used with permission. Information is correct at the time of going to press. Please visit the GDC web site to check for any changes since publication: www.gdc-uk.org (accessed 10 November 2015).

1 ECDBA

Option A and Option B are both inappropriate actions and therefore ranked fifth and fourth respectively. Ignoring the situation will be least helpful as it means no action is taken to resolve the problem. This is not the first time you have heard the receptionist speaking negatively about the clinical staff and therefore ignoring the situation at this stage will make it worse and could affect many more patients, staff members and the overall reputation of the practice. Whilst option B is stopping the receptionist's action, it is unprofessional to confront the receptionist in front of the patient and is more likely to result in a further confrontation. The conversation has also moved on, so intervening immediately will have little value.

Option E is ranked first. Your educational supervisor is usually your first point of call when dealing with tricky situations such as these and, as a more experienced member of the team, he/she will be in an ideal position to provide you with the best advice on how to deal with the situation. This may be your educational supervisor simply asking you to speak with the receptionist at an appropriate time or speaking to the receptionist himself regarding the situation on your behalf. Option C is ranked second as you are giving the receptionist a chance to explain her comments. At the end of the day, when things are less busy, you can use this opportunity to remind her about the importance of professionalism in front of patients and talk to her about any genuine concerns she may have regarding the clinical staff. Option C is ranked third, as the situation is more official; whilst reporting the receptionist to the practice manager may resolve things it will also involve escalating the situation to a level where the practice manager will have to officially reprimand the receptionist as a report has been made by you.

2   EDBAC

Option C is ranked last because, although working more may enhance your clinical experience, you will be officially breaking your legal contractual agreement with the deanery. Although reporting your educational supervisor to the GDC may seem excessive, it is not breaking your legal contracted hours and hence is ranked second last. The remaining three options all will provide viable solutions for you to deal with the situation appropriately.

Option E is ranked first. Should practices require them to do so, DFTs must work Saturdays as long as they are not working more than their weekly contracted hours. Option E is therefore most suitable as you will be given a regular day off during the week, thus not going over your contracted hours. You are also being a flexible team member and will expose yourself to different types of patients who can only be seen on weekends, which will be good for your experience. Option D is ranked second as your scheme leader knows all the information regarding working hours for DFTs and is most likely going to advise you and your educational supervisor to either allow you to work Saturdays and have another day off or politely say 'no' if no alternative day is being given off as it is breaking your working contract, which you and your educational supervisor and the deanery have agreed to.

3   DEBAC

This question is focusing on patient confidentiality. Patient confidentiality should not be breached unless there are exceptional circumstances. In this situation the patient's confidentiality should be maintained and therefore both option C and A are ranked last and second last. Although both options break confidentiality, option C is ranked lower then option A because it uses medical jargon terms and does not provide any other explanations.

The remaining options all respect patient confidentiality. Option A is ranked first as it is directly addressing the situation and providing the patients daughter with a reason as to why you cannot divulge the information to her. Both options E and B are potential solutions to the daughter's question, with option E being more suitable as you will be able to provide both patient and daughter with the most suitable information and advice.

4 ECDBA

Option E is ranked first as you are considering both patients by taking direct care of the patient who requires urgent medical attention and by notifying your next scheduled patient. Option C is involves the wider dental team, which is very important in a medical emergency situation. Option D is taking care of the patient; however, the patient may require treatment more urgently and may not be able to wait for an ambulance and therefore is ranked third best. Option B involves treating the patient in the waiting room. This is not an ideal place to treat the emergency. While the patient is still conscious it will be better for you to treat him in your surgery where you can lie him down and treat him privately, not in the middle of a busy waiting room. It is also not ideal leaving your nurse alone with your other patient in the surgery. Option A is ranked last as you are not placing patients best interest first.

5 EADBC

Your scheme leader would have dealt with many situations like this before and therefore is an ideal person from whom to seek advice. He will be able to assist you on how you can approach/speak to your educational supervisor, which may be difficult, especially as this is not the first time you feel your educational supervisor has been rude. Speaking with your educational supervisor at a suitable time will also most likely resolve the issue. Whilst you may find your educational supervisor to be undermining your work, it is always important to reflect on his comments and see if you can use them to learn from and improve your skills. Discussing your educational supervisor's action with the receptionist is very unlikely to help with the situation and ignoring it altogether and behaving normally will only make it worse.

6 ECDBA

By informing the parties involved, you are showing commitment to the profession and complying by the ninth GDC standard of ensuring you put professionalism first. Of course it is not a requirement to attend, as the meeting has just been arranged; however, it shows good faith by showing you are willing to attend if completely necessary. Therefore E comes first and C second as C suggests you are not putting a plan in action for catching up with the meeting. D is extreme; however, if the meeting is important – for example if a complaint has been made and the team must discuss it immediately – then at least you are in attendance. B has a lot of flaws, especially if you are handing over responsibility to a third party. It shows a lack of teamwork – and miscommunication could occur with regard to your nonattendance. You should always ensure you handle your own actions and do not leave crucial decisions up to others. B is a cowardly way out and should be avoided if possible – especially as a foundation trainee. A is unprofessional and shows a lack of respect for the team.

7 CADBE

Option C provides an opportunity for the nurse to explain his timekeeping issues with you, which may resolve the situation. The nurse will appreciate you speaking to him first before escalating the issue, especially as you have had a good working relationship with him in the past. Option A is the next logical action you would take if you could not speak to the nurse yourself. Your educational supervisor, as a more experienced colleague, can provide you with advice on how to approach your nurse. Your practice manager is there to deal with such issues and is in a position to help/reprimand the nurse without involving you thereafter. Option D is ranked third, although it may resolve the situation, it is not best practice to threaten the nurse with a complaint about him, making options C and A more suitable. Discussing the issue with associate dentists is least likely to resolve the issue. Option E is ranked last as this is not a GDC issue and needs to be dealt with in house.

8 BCDEA

Your educational supervisor is there to guide and assist your transition to seeing more patients safely therefore making option B your first choice. Seeing more patients gradually will improve your time management and give you the confidence to see more patients in a shorter time frame without compromising safety. Option C is ensuring no patients are placed at risk; however it does restrict your development as a FD. Option D may provide you with some good tips; however, your educational supervisor is in the best position to advise you on how to improve as he/she is working with you daily. The remaining options don't help the situation, Option E will add more pressure on your colleagues and limit your development as an FD, whereas option A could lead to compromising patient safety.

9 BCDAE

Option E is ranked last, as treating patients without your nurse is dangerous and not in the best interest of the patient or the clinician. Option A is ranked fourth because this option is not going to resolve the situation and is most likely going to make things worse. Forcing your nurse will not be helpful as her request for finishing work on time is reasonable. Similarly, option D, making a complaint about her, will not resolve the situation as she has not done anything wrong. The problem in this question is not the nurse's behaviour – rather, it is a time-management issue, which is either to do with the FD's patient time management or unreasonable appointment times booked in by the receptionists. Both options B and C will resolve the problem. From a FD's development perspective, option B is the first-ranked choice as your educational supervisor is in a perfect position to identify if the problem is with your patient time management or if the late afternoon appointment times for the treatment required are unreasonable, in which case option C is the next best answer.

10 BDCAE

Option B is ranked first. Your colleague has informed you about something personal and needs your support. You are giving him the opportunity to fix the matter himself. As a dentist and a colleague it is your duty to help your colleague; however, you must also keep a balance between helping your colleague and ensuring that no patients are harmed by his actions and therefore warning him that you will have no choice but to report him will cause him to act urgently himself. Your indemnity provider will provide you with advice on what you can do and the legal standpoint and obligation for both you and your colleague. It will also be able to direct you and provide you with information on support services, which you can pass on to your colleague.

Whilst option C is betraying your colleague's trust, it is the next best option you would take after first giving him an opportunity to address the situation himself and gaining all the information and advice on the matter you need from your indemnity provider. Only reporting your colleague after reviewing his skills is potentially unsafe. His clinical skills may have been safe on that study day but his future/past performances in practice may put patient's safety at risk.

Option E is ranked last as this will compromise patient safety. You cannot ignore the issue and hope that your colleague will overcome his addiction. He may have already caused harm to patients and may cause further harm if he is practising under the influence of cannabis.

11 CBEDA

Standard 7.1 of the GDC Standards for the Dental Team states: 'You must provide good quality care based on current evidence and authoritative guidance.'

General Dental Council prescribing guidelines state: 'Prescribing medicines is an integral aspect of many treatment plans. You must make an appropriate assessment of your patient's condition, prescribe within your competence and keep accurate records. Part of prescribing medicines responsibly means prescribing only where you are able to form an objective view of your patient's health and clinical needs.'

Without examining the patient you are unable to form an objective view of the patient's health and clinical need, therefore option A is ranked last as it is potentially putting the patient at risk. Without examining the patient you cannot be certain that he requires antibiotics. Option C is ranked as the best option as all parties in the situation are looked after. You are being a good team member to your nurse and putting the patient's interest first by agreeing to see him at a time convenient for him, thus allowing you to decide if he does require a course of antibiotics. Your nurse should not be diagnosing, even if the patient is her husband. She may feel she knows the cause for her husband's swelling but it's not within her remit and scope of practice to make a diagnosis and could put patients at risk. Prescribing medication without ever examining the patient is against prescribing guidelines. Option D is ranked fourth as you are not dealing with situation yourself and passing it on; however, it is not ranked last as you are not harming the patient by prescribing blindly.

12 AECDB
In a situation like this it is important that a senior member of the team is notified straight away. As a FD your educational supervisor is the most suitable person to inform and they will be able to advise you and others in the practice as to what has happened. Pretending not to realize and continuing with your day as normal is incompetent and can be potentially putting patients at risk. If the prescription pad has been stolen, nonprescribers could potentially prescribe harmful substances to themselves and others, thus making option B ranked last. Notifying your CCG is important as they can inform all local pharmacies not to dispense any prescriptions from the pad that is missing. Your indemnity provider will provide you with important advice on how to record and deal with the situation from a legal standpoint. Options A, E and C are all options that can/will prevent any further escalation to the problem and anyone coming to harm from the situation. Option D is ranked fourth as questioning your nurse should only come after all the preventative options have been taken.

13 DABCE
Informing your educational supervisor of your concerns and making the effort to arrange a timetable for him will most likely resolve the issue. It is important you speak to your educational supervisor, giving him the chance to address your concerns appropriately and fulfil his duty as a educational supervisor. If this does not resolve the issue the next logical step would be to speak to your patch associate dean, who is in an ideal position to speak to your educational supervisor regarding tutorials and any ePDP issues. A reminder from the patch associate dean should cause the educational supervisor to catch up on tutorials with more urgency.

Out of the remaining options (BCE), answer B is the next best option. Although it may not be ideal, as this is not the first time you have expressed these concerns to your educational supervisor, it is still better to trust your educational supervisor's judgment compared to option C and E. Your educational supervisors all know that they must complete a certain number of tutorials throughout the year. Whilst they should do one every week, there may be circumstances where tutors need to catch up on some tutorials.

Options C and E will not resolve the problem. It is not the responsibility of an associate to provide you with tutorials. Your educational supervisor is the experience teacher and has signed and agreed to a contract to provide you with all the tutorials throughout the year.

This is not really an issue for the GDC and is more suited to be dealt with by the deanery. Going to the GDC is escalating the situation to an unnecessary level.

14 DCEAB

Option D,C and E are all in the best interest of the patient. In all these options you are not placing the patient at any risk as you are either doing a different treatment you are confident with or being supervised by another dentist or the patient is being treated by another dentist instead. Option D is ranked first as it is better for the patient to be treated by the same dentist through a treatment plan and your educational supervisor is the most suitable dentist in the practice to observe you and guide you through the difficult procedure as they have/will be mentoring you through the year. In the cases where your educational supervisor is not available and another dentist is willing to guide you through the procedure before, during and after, then this is acceptable. Asking another dentist to treat the patient may benefit the patient but will not build on your development. If the option is available where you can carry out the treatment at a later date without affecting patient safety then it is better for you as a learning FD. All three options will improve the patient's oral health.

The two remaining options are not in the best interest of the patient. Option B can be potentially dangerous to the patients as you are carrying out a tricky procedure, which you have never done before and is therefore ranked last. Option A is inconveniencing the patient and is unprofessional, cancelling patient appointments when it can be avoided.

15 BECDA

This is a violation of the trainer-trainee contract. Your educational supervisor has to spend a minimum of 3 full days with you in a working week. In this situation it is best first to address your concerns to your educational supervisor. Reminding him of his contractual agreement and telling him you feel you are not getting the right amount of supervision is the first thing you should do. Your practice manager is someone you will see on a regular basis and therefore it is also a good option to seek advice from him. He is in a good position to speak to your educational supervisor, reminding him of his contractual and teaching obligation to you, allowing for the situation to be resolved within the practice. Option C is taking the situation further but may be a necessary step to take. Your scheme leader has regular reviews with all the educational supervisors and therefore will support you and address your concerns directly to the educational supervisor.

It is not the responsibility of the associates to provide you with supervision and guidance. There may be odd days and occasions where your educational supervisor is off on sick/annual leave where he may ask another dentist to assist in supervising the FD when required; however, this should only be an option in exceptional circumstances. Option A is not dealing with your concerns and the situation. In the question it is only your first month as a FD a time where supervision and guidance from your educational supervisor is most important. Continuing to practice as normal will harm your development and potentially put patients at risk.

16 CEDAB

Patient confidentiality is a GDC standard that all members of the dental team must adhere to and respect. Regardless of who the patient is, confidentiality should be respected at all times and the conversation should be stopped immediately. Option C is ranked first as it is addressing both members of the team who are involved in breaching confidentiality. Option E is only addressing your nurse and is therefore ranked second. Out of the remaining options, only option D is still acting against the situation. Although reporting the nurses to the principal will escalate the situation, the principal will reinforce the importance of maintaining the highest professional standards for the practice including patient confidentiality. Both options A and B are not acknowledging the breach in confidentiality; option B is ranked last as you are also breaching patient confidentiality.

17 DCBEA

Not only are options E and A inappropriate and unprofessional but they are also potentially placing patients at risk. If you drink a large (250 ml) glass of wine, your body takes, on average, about 3 hours to break down the alcohol. If you have a few drinks during a night out, it can take many hours for the alcohol to leave your body. The alcohol could still be in your blood the next day. The NHS advises people not to drive the next day after a heavy night of drinking as you could still be over the legal limit. It would therefore be very irresponsible of you, as a healthcare professional, to agree to treat patients the next day, even if it is after lunch especially as you have consumed a large amount of alcohol, therefore options E and A are ranked fifth and fourth.

The remaining options do not put any patients at risk and are more about how honest and professional you want to be with regard to your educational supervisor's request.

18 CDEAB

The patient must come first in this situation. Therefore alleviating the patient's pain is paramount; however, the issue regarding your associate not taking bitewings must also be addressed. Option C is ranked first, as the patient's symptoms are taken care of, putting the patient's interest first and then approaching the associate directly to enquire about the lack of bitewings. You should give the associate a chance to explain why he did not take any bitewings. It is important you inform a senior dentist regarding the associate's action, especially if you feel a patient has been affected as it is important to address the situation because many more patients may also be at risk.

Options E and A are ranked third and fourth respectively as, although they are dealing with the patients complaint, you are not following up on as to why the associate is not taking routine bitewing radiographs.

Asking the patient why no bitewings were taken isn't going to help too much with the situation. Most patients don't know when or why radiographs need to be taken therefore option B is ranked last.

19 DBCEA
Option A is not in the best interest of the patient. Although the parents are not present and consent is an issue, you should always act in the patient's best interest first. The remaining options all provide some form of treatment to the patient. Option E is the lowest ranked out of the remaining options as the patient has presented to you and you cannot be sure if the patients will go to the local specialist down the road. Options D and B are both in the best interest of the patient; however, due to the nature of the treatment it would be better for the patient and you as a learning FD to have the help of your educational supervisor, a more experienced dentist who has seen more cases like these. You will also be able to have a second opinion from your educational supervisor on the consent issue. You can then write in your notes that you and your educational supervisor agreed that it was in the best interest of the patient to proceed with treating the child. Option C is ranked after D and B because, although the child has a cavity that requires stabilization, the patient has come in to see you for the emergency trauma. It would be better for you to inform the patient and his brother of the additional cavity that you have seen and to make an appointment for that as soon as possible when the child's parents can also attend.

20 ACBED
Carrying out the treatment without local anaesthetic is definitely the worst option. The patient is already anxious and worried about pain. Carrying out the treatment without local anaesthetic is almost certainly going to cause her more pain and increase her anxieties further. As the patient is extremely needle phobic the option of carrying out the treatment under sedation should always be offered first. Although this may cost the patient more, or make her treatment take longer, the patient should be presented with all options first. The remaining options are all carrying out the treatment with the use of local anaesthetic but with differences in techniques. It is well known that injecting slowly causes less pain for the patient and using topical gel will also reduce the pain from the local-anaesthetic needle.

21 BDECA

All GDC registered members of the dental team are responsible for completing their own mandatory CPD. Your nurses are missing out on core training required for them to do their job to the highest required standards, which could potentially place patients and other colleagues at risk. Your practice manager is there to check all clinical staff members within the practice are up to date on CPD and therefore he/she is an ideal person to speak to the nursing staff. Showing your nurses the practice policy on CPD and raising CPD issues in a practice meeting will highlight to the nurses that you are aware of their situation, that what they are doing is wrong and that it could jeopardize their career and harm patients/colleagues. Option C is quite an extreme step to take initially and is therefore ranked fourth. If your nurses have not changed after making them aware that what they are doing is wrong then you will be left with no choice but to whistleblow. Options BDE and C will all cause the nurses to change their actions. Option A is ranked last as ignoring the situation will most likely not change the nurse's action, therefore potentially putting others at risk.

22 ADCBE

This question concerns your professionalism. Option E is ranked last. Deciding not to go in as you think most of your patients will cancel is very unprofessional. Regardless of whether you feel your patients will cancel, you should never just decide not to go in, especially without notifying your practice. Your receptionist will be the best person to contact. You are notifying the practice that you will have some difficulty getting in and will be late. This will give the reception staff an opportunity to call patients before their appointments to let them know of the delay. It also allows the reception staff to inform you if any patients have cancelled due to the weather, potentially giving you more time to commute. Your educational supervisor is also someone you should notify. He/she is probably in a similar situation and may be able to provide you with some assistance for your commute or help by seeing some of your patients if you are late. Although option C is not ideal, by cancelling the morning patients at least you are still making the effort to come in. It is still a better option than B and E.

23 BACDE

Social media can have a very large impact on the reputation of one's practice. It is very important how they are used. Clearly in this situation they are being used inappropriately and the first and foremost thing to do would be to delete any harmful/inappropriate comments. As an FD you will most likely not have access to the Facebook account; however, the practice manager should be made aware so she can delete the content accordingly. Once the content has been deleted, it is equally important that incidents like these do not occur again and therefore raising the issue in a meeting can hopefully ensure that there is no reoccurrence. Your indemnity provider will be able to provide you with some advice on what to do but will most likely tell you to ensure the content is removed as soon as possible. Keeping a log of all the events in your ePDP is a good thing to do as it will act as evidence that you did act in this situation should the incident be taken further. Option E is ranked last – the damage may already have been done, and turning a blind eye until next time may well be too late.

24 DACEB

Reassuring the patients that they will all be seen and asking for help is a good start to resolving this situation. All three patients require treatment – it is important you prioritize their needs. Ronny and Mrs Jones have treatment needs that are time dependent. Although Mr Smith has serious symptoms (swollen face) his treatment is not as urgent as a reimplantation and a bleeding patient. As you are only 3 weeks into your DFT year, it will be better to ask a senior colleague to treat Ronny and for you to take care of Mrs Jones whom you treated this morning. The remaining options are showing neglect towards the patients and are ranked according to the severity of neglect. In option B, all three patients are neglected and therefore ranked last. Choosing to treat one patient based on how easy that patient would be to treat is unethical and not in the best interest of the patient. As mentioned before, patients should be prioritized in accordance to their treatment needs.

25 ACBED

The patient is demanding treatment that is not in the best interest of her oral health. Regardless of whether a patient wants a particular treatment, if you feel it's not in her best interest it is important that you explain to the patient why you don't think she should have the treatment, fully justifying your answers and offering alternative, more feasible options that may still deal with her primary complaints. Option A is therefore ranked first. At times patients can be very demanding and in such situations a second opinion from another dentist can help the patient to understand. Your educational supervisor is ideal for this during your FD year. Option D is ranked last as you are carrying out treatment that is not in the best interest of the patient. Referring the patient to a specialist is not turning the patient away completely as you are still offering the patient an alternative treatment pathway. The remaining options are not in the best interest of the patient. Not offering any explanations and discharging the patient is neglecting the patient. Carrying out the treatment because the patient is persisting is ranked last as it will cause harm to healthy tooth tissue and worsen the patient's oral health.

26 BECDA

Although you are no longer in a university environment, it is important to remember that you are still learning and developing your skills during your DFT year. Therefore you should never feel foolish or incapable, especially on your first day. Hence option A is ranked last. Informing your educational supervisor and adjusting your patients is the best option, if this cannot be achieved then ensuring your educational supervisor helps you though out the treatment should allow you to complete the treatment in time. It is reasonable to ask your educational supervisor to help you through difficult appointments, especially early on in your DFT year. Option C is ranked third as it is a measure to prevent further situations like this and is therefore ranked after options B and E.

27 BCEAD

Option B is ranked first as the patient in the chair is your priority. He needs to be informed that your treatment will take longer than originally anticipated. Option C is ranked second as it is takes care of your next patient and makes him aware that you are running late. Informing reception not to book patients in catch-up slots will allow you catch up with your appointment times. Asking a free colleague to see Mr Smith may resolve the situation but only if the patient is happy to see another dentist. It is best that you treat your own patients as you would have built a rapport with them and would know their history best. Option D is ranked last – rushing through treatment is not in the best interests of the patient and can be dangerous. It is better for you to complete treatment safely and be late than rush through it and be unsafe. Option A is safer than option D; however, it is still unprofessional to assume that your next patient will be late and not to make your patients aware that you are running late.

28 EACDB

Options E and A, are ranked first and second as they are dealing with the immediate situation. If a patient has made a complaint it is part of the GDC standards to acknowledge the complaint and issue an apology. Reassuring patients that the event took place 2 days ago should ease their concerns. If no patient complaint was involved then option A is the next best option. Option C is ranked third best. No one expects you to be an angel but your behaviour in your private life can have an impact upon your professional life, causing immediate stress. Being more careful will prevent any such situation occurring again. The problem is with the photographs and they need to be removed as soon as possible. Option B is ranked last as threatening to sue is quite an extreme and expensive action to take and the problem can be solved more quickly and appropriately by asking for the pictures to be removed.

29 BDCEA

Option B is acting in the patient's best interest. Making sure that the whole mouth is healthy is paramount before proceeding to any aesthetic whitening treatment. Patients should clearly understand the risks of not having a healthy mouth in any treatment option and a clear written estimate for the whole treatment plan will cover all risks and benefits, informing the patient. Option A is likely to cause harm to the patient as his cavities and oral hygiene should be your primary concern. Whilst your opinion may not matter to the patient, it is still better than going ahead with the treatment. Referring the patient to a colleague is not directly harming the patient; however, it is your duty of care to the patient to treat his cavities and oral hygiene concerns as long as you feel it is within your remit.

30 DECBA

Option D is ranked first. Medical notes are legal documents and need to reflect true, contemporaneous information. While you appreciate confidentiality in this case, your notes should be as you would write them for any other patient. This is clearly a sensitive issue for the patient and as a new dentist you may not have come across it before. It is therefore a good idea to ask your educational supervisor for help. Your educational supervisor, being a more experienced dentist, will not only be able to reassure the patient better but will also teach you how to deal with such situations. Your indemnity provider will reconfirm to you that all notes need to reflect true contemporaneous information; however, C is ranked third as it is quicker, easier and more practical to inform the patient yourself or to ask your educational supervisor to assist you. Option B is not in the best interest of the patient and is very unprofessional. Eliminating all traces from the notes is illegal and hence ranked last.

31 CDBEA

The whole group is revealing confidential patient details and is acting unprofessionally. Informing the group that its behaviour is inappropriate should stop the conversation and prevent any such future breaches. The practice manager should be told so that he can take over the responsibility as breaches in confidentiality are taken very seriously. They are in the best position to speak to the nursing staff involved and take any further action accordingly. Option E is inappropriate at this stage as, although your indemnity provider will provide you with good advice, this will take time and is not practical. You need to deal with the situation as it is happening. Ignoring the situation is unprofessional and hence is ranked last. Option B is ranked third best. If you are not able to speak to all parties involved, then sometimes speaking to one of the individuals may enable that person to stop the others from behaving in this way. You are still acting as the situation is occurring, unlike in options E and A.

32 CBDEA

This is clearly unprofessional behaviour on the part of the nurse and she should be stopped immediately, making option C your best option. The practice manager should be told as this may have happened before and the practice is already aware of the situation. Speaking to your defence union will reinforce the above. Asking the nurse if she has done this before is relying on her to be honest and does not directly stop the current situation. Option A is ignoring the situation and is unprofessional and unsafe.

33 DBCAE

Option D is ranked first as this is a situation that you would have not encountered before. The information needs to be released as it is in the patient's best interest hence B is ranked second. The practice should have a clear, written practice protocol regarding safeguarding issues. The practice manager is well placed to start the procedure and your defence union will also help and reassure you. You need to share the information with social services but it is not your job to judge what social services should do. There are exceptional circumstances in which you will have to breach patient confidentiality, especially if you feel that it is in the best interest of the patient. Option E is ranked last because if you do nothing you place the vulnerable person in continuing danger.

34 CABDE

Your colleague may be distressed and will need help and support. However, the patient also needs attention and option C is the clear option as everyone is looked after, followed by option A and B. Your colleague should call his defence organization after the patient has been attended to and a full report should be made in the incident book. Option E is unprofessional and is not supporting your team.

35 ABDCE

It is important that you ask your educational supervisor for a second opinion on the patient's injuries. Your educational supervisor will be able to offer suitable advice on the severity of the injuries and whether he also feels there may be a safeguarding issue. It is also therefore very important all the injuries are recorded. Speaking to social services directly will help you with whatever further steps you need to take, if any, and your indemnity provider will also provide you with advice on where you stand from a legal point of view in regards to patient confidentiality and speaking with the child's parents. Whilst it is important to reflect on such cases, to learn from it is ranked last as reflection should only occur after the immediate situation is dealt with appropriately.

36 EBDAC

Your educational supervisor should be made aware if you are having any difficulties during your foundation year. Your educational supervisor may not realize that you are struggling with the new trainee nurse and therefore it is important to raise this concern with him. Your educational supervisor should be able to provide you with a more experienced nurse or arrange a schedule where you are not in charge of training the new nurse every day. If you feel you can't approach your educational supervisor then the best person to approach would be your TPD. Reflecting upon this in your ePDP will give you a good idea of how you are progressing working with the trainee nurse. You may find, in a few weeks, that you are managing fine. If you are still struggling you will then be able to show your educational supervisor your ePDP reflection, showing him that you have tried your best to work with and train the new nurse but that you are still struggling. Your ePDP reflection should ensure that your educational supervisor acts and makes the situation more manageable for you. It is important that you are continually progressing throughout your DFT year and therefore it does matter if you are running behind. It will hold back your development and experience as a new foundation dentist. Insisting that your nurse is changed at a team meeting may have the desired result; however, it is not working as part of a team and the other options are a more professional way of dealing with the situation.

37 BCDAE

If you have concerns regarding working standards especially something as serious as infection control, you should bring them to the attention of a senior member of staff and ensure that they are acted upon accordingly. It is always good to carry out an audit to see where the current standards are and how they can be improved. Making a note of all the infection-control issues is another way to highlight any substandard practices occurring within the clinic. Issues regarding infection control should be highlighted to everyone working within the practice and a practice meeting is ideal for this. If the other dentists also agree, the principal will need to act and provide some suitable CPD training. Infection control is a core mandatory CPD subject that must be studied yearly. Option E is ranked last – although you are ensuring you are washing your hands correctly, it is important that you raise the issue with a senior member of staff within the practice.

38 ABCDE

It is important to explain to the patient which treatments are available on the NHS as many patients are not aware of this. White fillings are available on the NHS – however, not for the purpose of aesthetic treatment. Sometimes you can face situations where it is difficult to decide if the treatment can fall under the NHS and therefore speaking to your educational supervisor for further guidance will help you decide and justify which treatments are suitable for NHS or private treatment. Offering the patient a referral to another dentist will more than likely pose the same issue for another dentist; however, you have at least offered the patient a suitable treatment options under the NHS and a referral if she wants to be treated elsewhere. Option D is acing unprofessionally as treatment should not be carried out for your own personal benefit. Option E is quite extreme and unrealistic – you will face patients with high expectations in any practice.

39 ADECB

Option A is the right thing to do. Claiming false CPD hours is very unprofessional, ranking option B last. It is good to inform the CPD training providers of the error as they may have sent out certificates to other delegates who also did not attend the course. It is important that you keep up to date with your CPD, rescheduling any missed sessions. This is a situation where, ethically, you should be inclined to do the right thing but if you are still in doubt on what to do your educational supervisor is a good person to speak to for further advice. He will also tell you to delete the certificate and reschedule the training. Options C and B are acting unprofessionally and going against the GDC standards.

40 BDCEA

Informing your educational supervisor that you have only carried out lab-based treatment when the clinical situation requires you to is the right thing to do. Your educational supervisor should not be prohibiting you from carrying out lab-based treatments based on the cost of his lab bill. Treatment should be offered and based on the best interest of the patients. You should therefore not change the way you practice based on your educational supervisor's remarks. As this is not the first time your educational supervisor has said this to you it would be a good idea to speak to your TPD for advice. Your TPD is in a position to remind your educational supervisor as part of their educational supervisor contract they should not be imposing any restriction on your treatments based on lab bills and should resolve the situation. The three remaining options are all unsuitable; however, option A is ranked last as it is not offering your patients all treatment options in their best interest, which is a legal requirement. Option C is ranked second last as the situation should be dealt with more locally before reporting your educational supervisor to the GDC. Whilst option C is unsuitable it is still better than options E and A.

41 EDCBA

The child has revealed that he is being abused by his stepfather and you have noticed bruising injuries during your examination. It is evident that the child's wellbeing is at risk at home and therefore you need to raise a concern and speak to the children safeguarding lead and child services. If you do not do this you are potentially putting the patient's life at risk. Option E is ranked first – it is important that your nurse stays with the patient and that you speak to both your educational supervisor and the safeguarding lead in your practice. Option E is ranked above option D only because you have also liaised with the safeguarding lead who is the most appropriate person to speak to in this situation as he is fully aware of what procedures to follow. Your indemnity provider will provide you with advice on how to approach and document the situation; however, this should be done after speaking to your educational supervisor/safeguarding lead. Leaving the responsibility with the mother to seek further help is putting the child at risk as you can't be sure if the mother will go and seek help as she may already be aware of the abuse and may not have acted upon it. Waiting to review in a week is putting the child's wellbeing at risk and may result him gaining more injuries, which could be avoided if you act on the situation immediately.

42 EACDB

Your receptionist may be in a difficult situation but it is important that she still acts professionally and respects all the rules. She would get into a lot of trouble by taking the money without authorized permission and therefore it is important you encourage her to put the money back and ensure she speaks to the practice manager regarding the incident. Option E is therefore the best option. The issue will need to be notified to a senior member of staff as this may not have been the first time that the receptionist has been taking money. Option E is the most considerate way and it will be better if the issue is first raised with the practice manager before the principal as she may already be aware of the situation and can act accordingly. Hence options C and A are ranked second and third respectively. Although you can bring up practice rules in a team meeting, it may still not make any senior staff members aware of the situation or prevent the receptionist from taking money again. Option B is ranked last as you are not acting morally and you are encouraging the receptionist's behaviour, which could lead both of you into trouble.

43 ADEBC

Options B and C are not in the best interest of the patient, option C being the worst as carrying out the treatment without taking a medical history could lead to the patient having incorrect treatment or treatment that could cause him further harm. Option A is ranked first as it is important that you inform the patient that it is in their best interest that they disclose their medical history before any treatment. Politely explaining why you require their medical history should solve the situation. Both options D and E are methods by which you can learn from such patient cases. Your educational supervisor and TPD tutor are more experience dentists who can teach you how to manage such patients. You will see your educational supervisor more regularly than your TPD and therefore option D is ranked above option E.

44 BDAEC

Your nurse may not be aware that she has to dry flush the chair at the end of the day. Showing her the proper chair set up and cleaning procedure should be enough to ensure infection control standards are met. Performing an infection-control audit will highlight a need for further training for all staff members in infection control, preventing any such issues occurring in the future. The practice manager can also arrange for staff to have further training in infection-control procedures and ensure everyone is confident and competent. Options E and C are impractical and time consuming. It is unlikely your principal will want to find a new nurse it is better to provide further training to the existing nurse.

45 EBCDA

If the lab has made a mistake with the shade and design of the bridge it would be good if lab staff can come and view the bridge at the time of the appointment. If it is clear the lab has made an error in the shade or the way it has designed it, labs are usually happy to make another one at no extra cost. This is why a good relationship between the clinician and the laboratory is necessary. As a foundation dentist it is necessary to call the laboratory and introduce yourself. Therefore option E is ranked first. Option A is ranked last. To assume that a patient will not mind the aesthetics as he is elderly is discriminatory against the patient. If there is an issue with shade from a professional standing then it is in the patient's best interest to adjust this for a good outcome. Informing the patient of all your concerns and gaining valid consent is the only way you can fit the bridge. Always keep the patient informed. If the patient is happy with the way the bridge looks and gives you consent to place the bridge, then the matter does not need to be taken further.

46 ADCBE

Regardless how trivial you feel the matter is, your educational supervisor is there to support and help you with all your clinical needs. Calling your educational supervisor or another available dentist to assist you will be in the best interest of the patient and will give you further experience in placing matrix bands on large molar teeth. Practicing placing matrix bands will ensure you are able to treat patients correctly. Auditing your matrix band placements will ensure you are continually implementing your skills. Option E is ranked last as it is not in the best interest of the patient.

47 BCDEA

Speaking to your educational supervisor is the best course of action to take. If your educational supervisor feels that the course will benefit your development and you provide the practice with enough notice, your educational supervisor should be able to reorganize your diary so you can attend the course in full but still fulfil your contracted hours. Your TPD will also more than likely advise you to speak to your educational supervisor/practice to see if you can have the day off as part of tutorials or CPD. If you are in a position where your practice is unable to give you an extra day off, your TPD may be able to arrange a study day or similar course for you if enough FDs were interested. Option D may be a suitable compromise as you are contracted for set annual leave. Whilst your foundation year is for you to learn the basics and get use to practice life, it is always important that you are proactive and attend courses that you're interested in and want to improve your skills on. Option A is ranked last as it is dishonest and unprofessional. You will be causing your fellow team members and patients unnecessary inconvenience and risk by calling in sick falsely.

48 CDEBA

Your patient is unhappy with the way your receptionist has communicated with him. It is important you address the patient's concerns and at the same time support your colleague. Apologizing to the patient and reassuring him is therefore ranked first. Both options D and E will address the situation to the receptionist who needs to be made aware of the patient's comment. Option D is ranked above E, as your receptionist is more like to be more receptive to a senior colleague. She may be unaware of how she is communicating with the patients. Calling in the receptionist immediately is likely to escalate the situation and laughing with the patient and ignoring the comment is not doing anything about the situation and therefore is ranked last. You must address the patient's concerns and make the receptionist aware of them in a professional manner, as her communication and behaviour will affect the practice's reputation amongst the patients.

49 CEDBA

As an FD, you would not have come across many situations like this before and therefore it will be best for you to consult your educational supervisor who can advise you accordingly. If the patient requires an official sick note for an absence of leave from university he should speak to his GP. You should only write what you feel is an accurate statement of the patient's condition and your clinical opinion as you would for your clinical notes. The remaining options are all writing a rest period more than your clinical judgement and therefore are ranked according to the time. Just because the patient is demanding you to write 4 weeks' rest does not mean you should go against your clinical opinion and therefore option A is ranked last.

50 AEDBC

You should not carry out complicated treatment that you have not done before unsupervised. If you discuss the case with the associate and he is willing to assist you then it is safe for you to go ahead with the treatment. If no one is there to supervise you it will be better for you and the patient to carry out other treatment that they require, with which you are more confident. Although cancelling patient appointments should be avoided, if a reasonable explanation is provided to the patient and appointment appropriately rescheduled, most patients are understanding. Option C is ranked last as it is not in the best interest of the patient. You have not carried out the treatment before and therefore it is in both the patient's and your interest that you are supervised/supported during the procedure. Although option B is unprofessional, it is not putting the patient at risk.

51 ADBCE

It is important that you record all information that you have found. Bringing the issue up in a team meeting is an appropriate platform as all members of the dental team will be present and therefore will be able to discuss the issue and how best to deal with it. Your educational supervisor will be a senior member of the practice and therefore will be able to arrange a meeting with the specialist practice. Although changing the specialist dental practice may resolve the issue, it may prove to be an inconvenience for patients as you may need to switch to a practice that is not as local and therefore it would be better to resolve the issue with the current specialist local practice. This is not a CQC issue and is also an extreme action to take, therefore option E is ranked last.

52 BDCEA

Your educational supervisor may already be aware of this issue and therefore seeking their advice on what to do with your patients is imperative. Your educational supervisor will be able to help you with all your extractions but also be able to speak to the oral surgeon directly to seek clarification as he is not putting the patient's best interest first. Similarly the raising concerns lead in the practice is usually a senior member of the team and will also be able to speak with the oral surgeon associate to resolve the issue. Whilst option C is not the quickest route for the patient, it still provides the patient with a pathway to be treated. The remaining options could result in a confrontation between you and the associate. It would be better if you dealt with the matter by asking your educational supervisor or another senior member of the team to approach the oral surgeon.

53 ADCEB

Mrs Jones will need a sympathetic and caring approach. Explain your findings and why it would not be in her best interest to go ahead with her request. Discuss all options with her and be supportive, not dismissive as in E. E is unprofessional and may be deemed negligent.

54 BCEDA

Mr S cannot understand English and is therefore unable to consent. The safety of any patient requires you to take a full and contemporaneous medical history. Mr S needs to be informed of this so his next of kin, Mrs S, could be approached by telephone and asked to explain. The nurse could also offer an explanation but in order to complete the work a translator should ideally be booked for the next visit if Mrs S cannot attend. Referring him to the in-house oral surgeon transfers the problem to a busy colleague. Taking the tooth out would be negligent.

55 DBCEA

This situation is a confidentiality issue. Regardless if she is the patient's wife, she will need to discuss with her husband the details of his dental appointment – therefore option D is ranked first. Both options E and A are breaches of confidentiality and against GDC guidelines. A is worse as you provide all the details. A senior colleague will reinforce and reassure you not to breach confidentiality regardless of how angry the wife sounds and B is therefore ranked second.

56 EBDCA

You are responsible for your own behaviour, as is your friend. Once you have encouraged him to leave, it is important that you think about yourself and therefore leave so that you feel safe to work tomorrow. Options C and A are the worst options. Option A is directly putting patients at risk. Regardless of how much caffeine you have during the day, having a late night whilst drinking can still affect your judgement and clinical work, placing your patients, your colleagues and yourself at risk. Although option C is extremely unprofessional and will cause inconvenience to your colleagues and some patients, it is not as bad as treating patients whilst being impaired.

57 DAECB

Your foundation year should concentrate on you developing your clinical skills and understanding of NHS dentistry, although private dentistry treatments will also greatly enhance your skills as a dentist with time and experience. Speaking with your educational supervisor should resolve the issue with the next best person to speak to being your TPD and practice manager. Option B is against your FD contract and is unprofessional.

58 BCADE

The question involves two issues – the clinical time-dependent procedure of reimplanting the tooth and obtaining a valid consent. It is in the patient's best interest to act immediately to allow the tooth to have the best prognosis. A senior dentist will have more experience in such cases and therefore is the first choice. Both options C and A involve the FD reimplanting the tooth; however, option C is ranked higher as it also incorporates a follow up with the child's parents to ensure they are aware of what occurred. Option E is ranked last. Although in this option consent will no longer be an issue, this will take the longest time and therefore gives the tooth a very poor prognosis, not being in the patient's best interest.

59 EABCD

This is a major concern and the dentists need to be informed quickly and promptly in regards to this scenario as E states. The next best answer is A, as you confront the nurse directly about her alcoholic smell. You need to assess the situation yourself and ensure that she is not fit to work and see if you can stop her from harming any patients or herself. Another nurse is needed, so you can call the company asking for another nurse and also informing it about the nurse's malpractice to ensure this never occurs again, as B suggests. C is an excellent statement; however, in terms of quick, short-term action, it does not handle the scenario as it stands and is more a factor to learn from with regard to the future. Training, meetings and peer reviews can all be done *after* the immediate management of the scenario. D is unprofessional and negligent with regard to the scenario at hand as you cannot dismiss the nurse's revelation on the locum nurse.

60 AEBDC

If you feel that your educational supervisor is teaching you out-of-date theory your TPD should be able to confirm this and speak to your educational supervisor to ensure that you are being taught based upon up-to-date literature and evidence. Dentistry is a dynamic ever-changing field; your educational supervisor may not be aware of new up-to-date theory and discussing new journals with him should make him aware of his shortcomings, ensuring that he makes sure he teaches you current theory. Writing your concerns on an ePDP is another good way for your educational supervisor and your TPD to notice that he is teaching you theory based on out-of-date literature. This is ranked third as it will take longer than options E and A. It is not the associate's job to teach you tutorials or your priority to arrange CPD for your educational supervisor and therefore ranked fourth and fifth.

61 DCBEA

The NHS FP17 form states that all treatment must be clinically justifiable and clinically necessary. Replacing amalgam fillings is not necessary – research shows longevity of amalgam fillings in posterior teeth and also a sound outcome. It can be presumed that the request to replace the fillings is for an aesthetic need, not a clinical need, so D is the first-ranked answer. As a FD, there are some areas you can learn from – educational supervisors will be able to shed light on this as C suggests. Examples where composites may be identified are very heavily broken down teeth where amalgam is not retentive, small fissure fillings, or buccal fillings – again where minimal invasion and retention may be an issue. B seems fair only if you are low on composites as an FD and the practice can accept a compromise. E is extreme as the patient is only asking and it's your professional duty to give the patients options. A is unethical. You should not be forging any clinical justification for treatment you carry out.

62 BCAED

Call for help as soon as possible, as B states. If you do not feel confident then do not continue on your own as it is not in the patient's best interest. The second best option is C, as the patient may need an experienced dentist to remove the roots – ensure, of course, that you give postoperative advice accordingly. A is not a bad answer, nor a great one as you are qualified, so fundamentally you do know what to do and have done one before; however, continuing depends on many factors, especially how confident you feel. If you do not feel confident then do not continue. E is the second last answer because, if you know that the patient needs surgical intervention then, by continuing with hand instruments and putting the patient and yourself through this ordeal, you are not going to gain anything and the patient may become frustrated and tired and this may even lead to complaints about your competence. Lastly, D is unethical and obviously not an option.

63 ACBDE

First and foremost, the nurse needs to register and understand the implications of her disclosure. The practice principal is the legal person who is liable for any issues that may occur in the practice – hence C is second priority. You can always call your educational supervisor for any advice and help, so C comes third. Never ignore the situation or dismiss the nurse's statement as this is unethical and negligent. D is a bad option in this situation as you cannot control this scenario on your own, especially as a foundation dentist – you need the support of the wider team, especially as this is a GDC legal requirement.

64 CABED

Being able to define your boundaries early on in your career will prevent you feeling overwhelmed. It is important that you are able to discuss these issues with your educational supervisor so that there is a clear understanding of what is expected of you. While this work is beneficial to the practice, the practice manager should be coordinating audits and policy-writing documents.

65 ABCDE

Your DFT year should be as stress free as possible. It is disheartening to discover that a educational supervisor is behaving in this way towards you as this is clearly counterproductive and will not help you as a trainee. Discuss the issues with the other educational supervisor and also your TPD and ask for a third party to intervene.

This will avoid any embarrassing conflict and help the educational supervisor understand what it is that is causing problems. Do not just put up with the behaviour as your focus will be taken away from DFT and you will become preoccupied with not wishing to attend!

66 ABEDC

This can sometimes happen when teeth are being extracted. An expression of consolation will do much to reassure the patient. It is important to ensure the safety of the patient so all procedures pertaining to the extraction procedure need to be adhered to. Invite the patient back the next day so that you can review the extraction site and make a decision as to whether it will be appropriate to recement the crown. In extremis, your educational supervisor can always be called to help explain the bad news.

67 ACDBE

The best solution is always to try and swap surgeries so that the treatment can be carried out. This is especially important when patients have taken time off work or travelled a long distance. An explanation is always reassuring and patients often understand and are often willing to have something else done so that it is not a wasted appointment. Using a hand scaler can provide the initial part of the treatment but if you know that the patient will have to return, this might be counterproductive. Solution B is extreme and E is unprofessional.

68 CDBAE

Without appropriate feedback, there can be no progress! Discuss the problem with your educational supervisor in the first instance and then approach the TPD for advice. Then feedback needs to be obtained from the assistant to enable you to move on with the audit. Discussing the issue with the practice manager could be useful as previous audits will show how these were done for the practice. However, it will not provide you with the information that you require to progress with your own audit. E is of limited use!

69 DBAEC

Problems of this nature should always be resolved through discussion. As a new trainee, it may be difficult to know to whom to turn for advice. Generally, a discussion among peers is a good starting point as it will help identify common problems. This, however, needs to be taken forward to the TPD so that you are able to explain your concerns and discuss options. A meeting between your educational supervisors and trainees with a mediator to discuss the issues at hand is recommended. E is counterproductive and C will not resolve the issue.

70 AECBD

Patient safety in practice is paramount. The actions of the nurse are unprofessional and could have huge repercussions for you and the practice. Signal to her to start mixing again with a new spatula and speak to her and to the head nurse afterwards as this is poor infection control. Asking for another nurse will not address the learning needs of the first nurse and shouting at any team member is totally unprofessional. Option D, while appearing to be kind, only condones her actions.

71 AECDB

The behaviour of the receptionist is unprofessional. She should be asked to leave so that you can complete the task in hand. If you have an agreed time to finish and you over run then you will need to be aware of the impact of your actions on other team members. If, however, you are within the agreed time, you should not feel pressurized to finish. Always be aware of the wider picture with the team. Does the receptionist have childcare issues? Discuss the issue with the practice manager so that he may discuss any potential, undisclosed problems.

72 ABDCE

Your year in DFT is pivotal in your future development as a GDP. The study days are meant to provide you with appropriate guidance on important issues. If this is not provided then you may carry unresolved problems with you into your career and this may have a negative impact on your performance. Action is required and concerns need to be expressed as a collective group. Seek advice from another TPD on a different scheme on what to do and also ask your educational supervisors collectively to speak with the TPD. Ignoring his behaviour condones his actions, which may ultimately affect you.

73 BCEAD

You have a legal duty to ensure that your health does not impact upon the treatment of your patients. Starting your career off with back problems does not bode well and could force you to retire earlier than you would wish. Ask your educational supervisor for tips and supervision on your posture and use of the mirror and also for a new chair so that your posture may be improved. Doing nothing will worsen the problem and shorten your career as a GDP.

74 CDEAB

Constructive criticism should not be confused with being insulted. Your nurse will have gained much experience throughout her career in communicating effectively with patients. Sometimes we need to take on board what our colleagues tell us, especially if it affects our patients. Asking your nurse to attend your next tutorial to discuss the issue with your educational supervisor is a good idea. Do not feel insulted as this will only make for poor relations between you and the nurse. It sounds as though she has your best interests at heart.

75 BADEC

Your TPD will be the source of signoffs and will be able to guide you in what has to be done and what guidelines to follow. If an extension can be provided to finish your clinical activity then your TPD will be the only one who can facilitate this. Secondly, your educational supervisors should be involved. They would be the standard everyday point of call to help you if you need to start finding bridge cases. The third option would be to compare with others on the scheme – it is good to keep in the loop in terms of what the others know about the guidelines. Ensure you have a good working relationship with the other FDs on your scheme. Doing nothing is not good but is better than lying about your clinical activity.

'Best of three' SJTs: Questions

Questions are from the General Dental Council, used with permission. Information is correct at the time of going to press. Please visit the GDC web site to check for any changes since publication: www.gdc-uk.org (accessed 10 November 2015).

1 A patient you treated in the morning has come back 10 minutes after leaving, complaining to you that some cash has disappeared from his coat pocket. The coat was placed on the hanging rail in your clinic by your nurse. While treating this patient you had to leave the room to attend to an emergency call from reception. Your nurse remained in the room with the patient.

   Choose the three most appropriate answers when all of the answers are considered together.

   a) Tell the patient he must have made a mistake, suggesting he may have lost the money after he left.

   b) Confront your nurse immediately as she was the only other person present in the room. Ask her to replace the money.

   c) Call the police.

   d) Ask the patient for details about the alleged theft, reassuring him that you will do what you can to deal with the issue. Notify the practice manager of the problem.

   e) Remind the patient that he should be more careful about his possessions and tell him that you will see what you can do.

   f) Send an email to all your colleagues notifying them of the incident and asking them to warn their patients to be careful with their personal possessions.

   g) Do nothing.

   h) Dismiss all comments from the patient and offer him a free hygiene clean.

2 A 10-year-old child attends with her teacher from school as an emergency patient after falling over in an accident in school netball, resulting in the complete avulsion of UL1. The teacher informs you the accident occurred 10 minutes ago and the tooth was immediately placed in a bottle with mineral water. The teacher informs you that the child's mum has been contacted but it will take at least 45 minutes for her to reach the practice from work. The child is feeling a little dizzy as she has not eaten all day but other than that she feels fine. What do you do?

   Choose the three most appropriate answers when all of the answers are considered together.

   a) Reassure the patient with glucose, place her in a supine position to help her recover from dizziness and wait for her mum to arrive before you commence any treatment.

   b) Reassure the patient, lay her down and reimplant the tooth.

   c) Advise the teacher to take the patient to the local accident and emergency department as she is showing signs of head injury.

d) Ask your educational supervisor for advice and a second opinion.

e) Refer the patient to the local specialist paediatric dentist down the road who is more equipped to treat her injuries.

f) Refuse to see the patient as she is not at an age to consent and you deem it inappropriate to regard the patient as Gillick competent as the patient is currently in shock.

g) Act in the best interest of the patient and reimplant her tooth as quickly as you can. Provide the patient with some glucose and gauze to take home with her and a leaflet with all the postoperative instructions.

h) Question the teacher on how the accident happened, as you want a thorough history.

3 Your educational supervisor asks you to make a backdated alteration to handwritten notes in order to cover up for a past mistake he made on a patient you treated in the morning.

Choose the three most appropriate answers when all of the answers are considered together.

a) Make the change requested by the educational supervisor as you are worried he may give you a bad reference if you refuse.

b) Refuse to make the entry.

c) Make a note of the conversation that you have had with the educational supervisor and speak to your indemnity provider.

d) Agree to make the change at the time but do not follow through with it and hope your educational supervisor does not find out.

e) Inform the patient of the mistake as he has a right to know.

f) Inform the police as there are potential legal complications.

g) Report your educational supervisor to a nurse.

h) Inform your educational supervisor that you don't feel comfortable and advise him to speak to the patient, informing him of the mistake.

4 Your DF1 educational supervisor is complaining about the bad body odour of your nurse and asks you to speak to her. You were aware of the problem before but found it difficult to raise it with the nurse.

Choose the three most appropriate answers when all of the answers are considered together.

a) Tell your educational supervisor that you don't feel comfortable speaking to the nurse and that he should do it himself.

b) Go out and buy a variety of deodorants and perfume as a gift for your nurse, informing her she has been a great help throughout the year and hope this will solve the problem subtly.

c) Raise the issue at the next team meeting in front of your nurse.

d) Email all the staff in the practice, asking them to drop hints subtly to the nurse she has a body-odour problem.

e) Speak to your nurse in private. Inform her of the issue and respectfully ask her if she has a medical problem and provide appropriate advice to help her deal with the problem.

f) Ask the practice manager to speak to the nurse.

g) Tell your nurse everyone has noticed it and she needs to improve her hygiene.

h) Send your nurse an anonymous note discussing the issue.

5 You are about to see a new patient. You ask your nurse to call him in but she refuses to work with you on this patient. She says she will return once you are finished. She leaves the surgery in a rush. You notice that the patient's medical history discloses he is HIV positive. What do you do?

Choose the three most appropriate answers when all of the answers are considered together.

a) Call the head nurse immediately for support in staffing arrangements.

b) Call your indemnity provider.

c) Speak to your educational supervisor, and suggest CPD for all clinical staff to reflect on this scenario.

d) Ask reception to ask your patient to be seated as you are running a few minutes late.

e) Ask the practice manager for the nurse to be fired.

f) Report the nurse to the GDC.

g) Ask to move training practices as you cannot work under this stress.

h) Call the patient in and begin treatment alone.

6 You are running the emergency clinic today and reception has called into your surgery stating that a young boy has arrived, with his grandma, hysterical and complaining of severe tooth pain. You see the young boy and diagnose an acute condition on his lower left molars. He is in severe pain and his grandmother insists you help them today, as his parents are both at work. What do you do?

Choose the three most appropriate answers when all of the answers are considered together.

a) Start treatment on both molar teeth, taking all relevant radiographs and doing special investigations. Advise the grandmother on what you have done and suggest a follow up with his parents.

b) Familiarize yourself with the children policy of the practice.

c) Do a full thorough examination and make contemporaneous notes then seek advice from your educational supervisor on how to proceed further.

d) Speak to your dental indemnity provider for informal advice on how to proceed.

e) Make a courtesy call to the child's mother and gain consent over the phone to be reiterated in writing when she can come into the practice – preferably within 24 hours.

f) Refuse to see the child and suggest that the grandmother call the emergency NHS dental hotline.

g) Go to the reception desk and explain that you cannot treat children without valid consent from their parents – that you will endeavour to do what you can but there are no guarantees.

h) Hang up on the reception staff after telling them they should know better than to ask you to treat patients illegally.

7 You start your DF1 induction in practice. You soon find out several of the dental nurses are not sterilizing all the equipment as best practice requires. You query why this is the case with the head nurse who replies that the educational supervisor does this to save on costs. What do you do?

Choose the three most appropriate answers when all of the answers are considered together.

a) Tell the head nurse that, for all patients, you require fully sterilized equipment to comply with CQC regulations and best practice.

b) Set up a meeting with your educational supervisor to discuss the matter and endeavour to make her comply with regulations.

c) Make a written formal complaint to the GDC for malpractice.

d) Contact your TPD to discuss this matter further insisting that he assist you further in your issue.

e) Contact your indemnity provider for informal advice.

f) Bring the issue up in a communal staff meeting highlighting the areas of concern.

g) Set up a meeting with your educational supervisor, practice manager and TPD to discuss this infection control issue and how uncomfortable you feel in this situation.

h) Report the practice to the CQC anonymously.

8 After the busy Christmas and New Year's period you find yourself very much behind with your ePDP. January is generally an extremely busy time and you are finding yourself stressed at how many patients you are seeing. The clinical and coursework load is getting too much for you to handle. What do you do?

Choose the three most appropriate answers when all of the answers are considered together.

a) Speak to your educational supervisor as soon as possible to tell him your issues and ask if time can be allocated for administrative work rather than clinical time.

b) Try to manage for as long as you can until your work starts affecting your patients.

c) Bring up your concern at a practice meeting, stating that reception staff are booking too many patients in for everyone.

d) Make a plan for the month to get back on track using evenings and weekends to do administrative work; show this to your educational supervisor for advice.

e) Ignore the ePDP for now. You can do it at the end of the month – all weekend if need be.

f) Speak to your personal TPD for advice on how you are feeling, suggesting he speak to your educational supervisor.

g) Speak to your colleagues, complaining all the way.

h) Tell your nurse that your New Year's resolution is to become more organized.

9 The trainee nurse you have been working with confides in you that the TePe brushes are being reused on patients. The nurse has been hired on a trial basis and is not doing very well. The nurse will probably be let go if you bring this to the practice principal's attention. What do you do?

Choose the three most appropriate answers when all of the answers are considered together.

a) Write down the incident and take to the practice principal in the hope that you can convince him that the nurse just needs further training.

b) Teach the trainee nurse about infection control in your spare time.

c) Tell the nurse this is not compliant with HTM01-05 and all TePe brushes are single use. Explain she must speak to the practice principal and not reuse them.

d) Speak to the practice principal with the infection control lead and explain the incident that occurred suggest trainee nurses gain further CPD in infection control.

e) Stress to your practice principal the importance of complying with CQC and best practice policies.

f) Ignore what the nurse says as she is only a trainee and assume that she does not know what she is talking about.

g) Familiarize yourself with the practice policy in infection control protocol and bring up the incident at a practice meeting.

h) Suggest to the practice manager that the trainee nurse is fired for malpractice.

10 You are in your first month of practice when you realize how overwhelmed you are with patients. You have 15 minutes, on average, with all patients from your first day, leaving you tired and making poor judgments on patients' treatment. It is also affecting your clinical work and you are finding yourself taking short cuts. What would you do?

Choose the three most appropriate answers when all of the answers are considered together.

a) Speak to reception and tell them the amount of time you require per treatment option.

b) Speak to your educational supervisor and ask her for suggestions on what to do.

c) Come up with a future plan that gives you time to build up on how many patients you see, the length of appointments and log your progress on ePDP.

d) Speak to your TPD for advice on the situation.

e) Speak to your TPD and ask to be moved to a different practice as you and your educational supervisor clearly are not suited.

f) Keep going as at some point you will be efficient enough to see patients in 15 minutes.

g) Start booking in fake patients in between real ones to give yourself the extra time at first.

h) Speak with your indemnity provider for advice.

11 The majority of your patients who are being treatment planned in the first quarter of DF1 have undiagnosed periodontal disease. Most are unaware what gum or periodontal disease is and claim to have never had a BPE and to have never been referred for hygiene appointments. What do you do?

Choose the three most appropriate answers when all of the answers are considered together.

a) Treat the patients at the standard that you are used to, highlighting their disease to them and putting treatment plans in place.

b) Treat the patient in line with what is best practice, ignoring the previous associate's malpractice.

c) Write to the GDC complaining about your colleagues.

d) Discretely bring this matter up with your educational supervisor and suggest CPD learning for the entire team.

e) Look for another job as you do not agree with this way of treating.

f) Call your indemnity provider for informal advice.

g) Familiarize yourself with the practice policy and meet with the raising concerns at work lead for the practice.

h) Encourage your patients to raise complaints.

12 You notice that your Friday afternoon patients continue to miss appointments. You investigate this further seeing that majority of these patients do not exist anymore or are new patients with no history. You come to the conclusion the support staff are creating patients so that they get to leave early on a Friday. What do you do?

Choose the three most appropriate answers when all of the answers are considered together.

a) Ignore this. You also want to leave early. If someone else is to blame, why stop them?

b) Discretely bring this up with the reception staff and warn them if this continues you will have to take this further.

c) Discreetly tell your educational supervisor, asking him to intervene and speak to the support staff about their malpractice.

d) Speak to the practice manager, asking her to fire the Friday receptionists.

e) Speak to your nurse asking if she can bring it up at a practice meeting.

f) Hold a meeting with your educational supervisor, practice manager and reception team to emphasize the importance of best practice, suggesting the reception gain more training.

g) Call your indemnity provider for informal advice.

h) Complain to CQC about the lack of training your practice principal has given the reception team.

13 You are seen at a local pub smoking socially on a Friday night. One of your patients comes over looking very angry, accusing you of being a hypocrite as you delivered smoking cessation to him previously that week. What do you do?

Choose the three most appropriate answers when all of the answers are considered together.

a) Try to calm him down, explaining that you are only a social smoker and the quantity probably will never affect you in the long run.

b) Tell him that this is not the time or place to be discussing confidential matters and suggest you see your patient on Monday morning to discuss this further.

c) Write up the incident and explain to your educational supervisor what occurred, asking for advice.

d) Call the patient on Monday giving him a month's free dental treatment for periodontal disease as an apology.

e) Try to speak discretely to your patient asking him to calm down or you will have to call the police for harassment.

f) Ignore the patient, pretending you do not know him, and deal with this another time.

g) Leave the pub, call your indemnity provider for informal advice and hold a meeting with your educational supervisor and practice manager on handling this complaint.

h) Tell him to do as you say, not as you do.

14 You walk into an associate's dental surgery midtreatment to ask for his help on a crown preparation that you are doing. You see him in a close embrace with his patient. Both look shocked and embarrassed to see you. What do you do?

Choose the three most appropriate answers when all of the answers are considered together.

a) Close the door, pretend you didn't see what you saw and carry on with your day, not mentioning this to anyone.

b) Report the couple to the CQC.

   c) Wait for an explanation. If it is valid and they are going to disclose their relationship then leave them to do it in their own time.

   d) Explain that you will now need to report this to the rest of the staff but will do this respectfully.

   e) Wait for an appropriate time to speak to the associate and ask for an explanation.

   f) Remind the associate of patients and dentists having an appropriate professional relationship.

   g) Speak to your educational supervisor for advice.

   h) Have a quiet word with the associate afterwards and tell him what a lucky fellow he is.

15 You overhear the dental nurses planning to use the radiograph room at lunch time to take radiographs of each other's teeth. What do you do?

   Choose the three most appropriate answers when all of the answers are considered together.

   a) Immediately stop them all; this is against GDC scope of practice and is illegal malpractice.

   b) Discretely walk past and pretend not to see anything as this is a very serious crime.

   c) Suggest, at the next practice meeting, that all dental nurses gain CPD in radiography and its hazards.

   d) Discretely stop the nurses. Tell them you will give them all an examination and prescribe them the radiographs in retrospect but tell them not to do it again.

   e) Report the incident to the practice manager and your educational supervisor.

   f) Suggest that nurses who want to broaden their scope should take radiography courses.

   g) Familiarize yourself with the policy for raising concerns and bring this incident up with the practice principal

   h) Report them to the GDC.

16 You overhear the reception team diagnosing patients at the front desk. It is a busy day and a few of the patients are getting carried away disclosing all their symptoms to the reception team. You overhear the head receptionist saying 'it is probably a root canal and you'll need some antibiotics' to your next patient. What do you do?

   Choose the three most appropriate answers when all of the answers are considered together.

   a) Call your patient through ignoring the receptionist and explaining the relevant treatment for your patient in the surgery.

   b) Call your patient through, telling him to ignore the reception staff and refrain from indulging in their symptoms in the waiting area.

c) Speak to the receptionist in front of the patient telling her to stop diagnosing patients in the waiting room, highlighting everything wrong with this.

d) Call your patient through but speak to the receptionist in private explaining that she cannot diagnose in the waiting room, especially as it is out of her scope and the issue of confidentiality.

e) Bring up the incident at a practice meeting.

f) Write up an incident form to hand into your educational supervisor and practice manager.

g) Suggest to the practice principal that the reception staff should be fired for their behaviour.

h) Suggest reception staff get extra training in patient management and what is within their scope.

17 You placed a preformed metal crown on a 6-year-old girl a few weeks ago. The patient and her mother attend your clinic with her mother complaining that the metal crown is extremely 'ugly' and would like it removed. She is adamant that the crown is taken off today or they will be moving dental practices. What do you do?

Choose the three most appropriate answers when all of the answers are considered together.

a) Sympathize with the mother, explaining that it is unfortunately a disadvantage and give her other options for her child's tooth and the consequences of these.

b) Ask for a second opinion from your educational supervisor and discuss options with the mother.

c) Ultimately, the metal crown is the best option and any other treatment is not in the patient's best interest so decline to take the crown out.

d) Try to communicate that you do not respond to threats and will do what is best for the patient disregarding her view about taking the crown out.

e) Refuse to treat the child due to the mother's threatening behaviour and discharge her from your care.

f) Write up an incident report from which the rest of the practice can learn at future meetings.

g) Reflect upon the tricky situation you were placed in today in your ePDP.

h) Ignore the mother and carry on with your work. After all, you are the professional.

18 You are in the middle of a surgical extraction when the receptionist walks into your surgery telling you discreetly that she has just received a patient complaint about you. What do you do?

Choose the three most appropriate answers when all of the answers are considered together.

a) The patient comes first. Stay focused and inform the receptionist that you will deal with it after you have completed treatment.

b) Ask an associate who is free to take over, fully explaining the patient history and go and deal with your complaint.

c) Continue with treatment and ask the receptionist for more details about the complaint.

d) Ask your educational supervisor for advice.

e) Tell your receptionist that she has put you in an awful position and has directly affected the patient's safety.

f) Call your indemnity provider for advice on how to deal with complaint.

g) Temporize the patient, apologize for not being able to complete the extraction and refer the patient to the oral surgery specialist.

h) Tell your receptionist to go away.

19 You are carrying out a routine restoration on your patient who said he's always a little anxious about dental treatment even though he has been through many treatments before. Your patient begins to breathe heavily and is complaining of pain from his chest. He goes on to say that he was having a dull ache earlier in the day but thought it was heartburn after having a heavy full English breakfast and he took some of his usual Gaviscon dose. You can see that the patient is becoming more restless and complains of dizziness. You see from his medical history that the patient is a type 2 diabetic, taking statins for his cholesterol and is on a variety of hypertensive medication.

Choose the three most appropriate answers when all of the answers are considered together.

a) Stop all treatment, sit the patient up and try to reassure him and help him get his breath back.

b) Stop all treatment, sit the patient up and administer GTN as you suspect patient is having an acute angina attack.

c) Ask your nurse to get you the salbutamol inhaler to help the patient with his breathing.

d) Stop all treatment, keep the patient in a supine position and administer GTN as you suspect patient is having an acute angina attack.

e) Carry on your treatment as you are close to finishing and hope that the patient's symptoms resolve.

f) Ask the nurse to call for an ambulance.

g) Ask your nurse to get the oxygen supply ready.

h) Call the wife of the patient to tell her to collect her husband after treatment.

20 On your study day, your DF1 colleague confides in you that his previous partner contacted him saying he has been diagnosed with HIV and may have had the virus whilst he was in a sexually active relationship with him. Your colleague is worried he may have contracted the virus also and needs your advice. He would appreciate that you keep the matter confidential.

Choose the three most appropriate answers when all of the answers are considered together.

a) Report your colleague to the GDC.

b) Advise your colleague to make an appointment with occupational health to get a checkup.

c) Advise your friend not to worry. The chances of transmission are still relatively low and he would have known by now if he had the virus.

d) Advise your colleague to contact his indemnity provider.

e) Advise your colleague to speak to his educational supervisor.

f) Advise your colleague that regulations have changed and dentists with HIV can still legally work so just book an appointment with his GP to get checked.

g) Advise you colleague to cancel all his patients and take sick leave until he has had a checkup from occupational health.

h) Seek advice from your indemnity provider.

21 You have been working with the senior practice nurse for the last three weeks. She is supposed to be more experienced than your previous nurse and is also trained to take radiographs. You find she wants to take all your radiographs and, upon developing, openly begins to diagnose the radiographs in front of the patient. Whilst most of the time she is not wrong, you are finding it inappropriate for her to interpret the radiographs in front of the patient, especially as there have been a few occasions where you disagree with her interpretation of the radiograph. What do you do?

Choose the three most appropriate answers when all of the answers are considered together.

a) Remind your nurse that it is not within her scope of practice to be interpreting and diagnosing from radiographs.

b) Inform the nurse that a diagnosis cannot be made from radiographs alone and that she should use a combination of history, examination findings and radiographs to come to the correct diagnosis.

c) Let it go, as you do not want to cause a scene with the senior nurse.

d) Ask your educational supervisor to give you a new nurse.

e) Ask your educational supervisor to speak with the senior nurse.

f) Report your nurse to the GDC.

g) Ask your indemnity providers for advice.

h) Tell the practice manager to explain politely to the nurse that she requires more mandatory CPD.

22 It is your first week in practice and you have been shadowing your educational supervisor and the principal dentist on a variety of treatments. You notice that neither uses a rubber dam when carrying out root-canal treatment, even when it has been clinically possible to do so. You have also noticed that there are no rubber dam sheets kept in the practice, with the head nurse informing you she does not order them because the dentists feel using a rubber dam is a waste of time and money. Your educational supervisor has said to you as long as your

nurse is suctioning properly you will not need to use a rubber dam for your patients requiring root-canal treatments. What do you do?

Choose the three most appropriate answers when all of the answers are considered together.

a) Accept this as practice policy and carry out your root-canal treatments without a rubber dam.
b) Ask your indemnity provider for advice.
c) Speak to your educational supervisor and say you are not comfortable doing root-canal treatments without a rubber dam. Ask for them to be ordered.
d) Remind both your educational supervisor and the principal dentist that not using a rubber dam is not putting the patient's best interest and safety first.
e) Do not carry out any root-canal treatments.
f) Ask your TPD for advice and assistance.
g) Report your educational supervisor to the deanery.
h) Advise the practice manager to order the rubber dams.

23 While compiling your DF1 audit project you notice a lot of the staff have not got the correct qualifications to nurse in the United Kingdom. You check the employer's folder and a lot of the CPD is either out of date too or nonexistent. What do you do?

Choose the three most appropriate answers when all of the answers are considered together.

a) Ask to speak to the practice manager highlighting the issue at hand.
b) Contact your TPD seeking further advice about your concerns and ask to be moved to a different practice.
c) Try to train up your nurse to your standards.
d) Familiarize yourself with the practice policy and follow protocol on how to raise this as a concern.
e) Omit these findings from your audit project.
f) Seek advice from your indemnity provider.
g) Take copies of all the nurses' qualifications and send them to the CQC as an anonymous complaint.
h) Suggest at a practice meeting that everyone should be compliant with their CPD and folders should be kept up to date.

24 Your nurse has been practicing for 15 years and tells you she is not registered with the GDC.

Choose the three most appropriate answers when all of the answers are considered together.

a) Explain the implications of her disclosure, encouraging her to register immediately.
b) Call your educational supervisor immediately and force the nurse to confess.
c) Call the GDC and disclose the nurse's statement.

d) Call an emergency practice meeting.

e) Speak to the practice principal immediately.

f) Log the nurse's confession and watch her closely.

g) Dismiss her confession.

h) Report her to the CQC.

25 A longstanding patient of the practice attends, enraged that his personal file was laid out on reception with a large red sticker on the front, which indicates that he has a 'high-risk' medical history. You notice that the patient is HIV positive. What do you do?

Choose the three most appropriate answers when all of the answers are considered together.

a) Stay calm, alert the reception and try to empathize with the patient.

b) Seek assistance from other members of the practice.

c) Bring this up at a practice meeting as soon as possible.

d) Keep an audit and reflect upon this in your ePDP.

e) Assure the patient this is not the case but indicate how he could complain.

f) Go out and tell the reception staff off for their tardy behaviour.

g) Offer the patient a goodwill appointment today.

h) Tell the patient to leave as you do not like his attitude.

26 You are in your first week of DF1 where an emergency session has been blocked off for you in your diary. You are seeing an 18-year-old girl who attends with pain localized to her upper second premolar. She has an associated abscess, which is confirmed by a radiograph you take, and she is complaining of soreness on biting. Ibuprofen has alleviated the pain but now she needs treatment. Your diagnosis is periapical periodontitis and after a discussion a decision is made to extirpate the tooth today with further visits for endodontic treatment. You have finished extirpation when you realize you have treated the upper first premolar, not the second! What do you do?

Choose the three most appropriate answers when all of the answers are considered together.

a) Start extirpating the second premolar and root canal the teeth together.

b) Call your educational supervisor in as soon as possible, asking for advice and where to go from here.

c) Call your indemnity provider for anonymous advice.

d) Write contemporaneous notes, explain to the patient what has occurred, apologize and highlight all options.

e) Explain to the patient what has occurred and show her the complaints protocol.

f) Ask your nurse to call your educational supervisor whilst you explain to the patient what has gone on.

g) Do an audit on your root-canal treatments, focusing on clinical ability.

h) Dress the tooth. Let the patient go and speak to your educational supervisor about what to do next.

27 You are in the middle of a molar RCT when you realize that there has been separation of the file that you have been using.

Choose the three most appropriate answers when all of the answers are considered together.

a) Carry on regardless even though you cannot see the instrument and assume that it will remove itself as you are shaping.

b) Assess whether the instrument is visible and remove it.

c) Stop because you cannot see the separated file and you need to make a radiographic assessment.

d) Temporize and tell the patient to come back next week.

e) Tell the patient to take ibuprofen.

f) Fully explain to the patient what has happened and offer an expression of consolation.

g) Explain what has happened to the patient and recommend a good endodontist.

h) Feel confident that all will be well in the end.

28 You notice that your nurse and receptionist are not getting on well and it has started to affect the atmosphere in the practice.

Choose the three most appropriate answers when all of the answers are considered together.

a) Tell them to grow up and behave.

b) Speak to them individually and tell them that you will send them each a disciplinary letter if their behaviour does not improve.

c) Keep them far away from each other at every possible opportunity.

d) Suggest a team-building day to your practice manager.

e) Suggest a meeting so that issues can be discussed openly and try to resolve the issues.

f) Inform your practice manager and ask her to intervene.

g) Recommend a psychotherapist.

h) Call your indemnity provider for advice.

29 You are coming to the end of your DFT year and are being shadowed by your replacement. You are very concerned about her unprofessional attitude and have received negative feedback from the dental team. She asks you to complete a feedback form for her dental school.

Choose the three most appropriate answers when all of the answers are considered together.

a) Politely tell the student throughout her placement that she should adjust her attitude.

b) Wait until the end of the placement and then meet somewhere privately to discuss your concerns.

c) Mark all the domains as, 'satisfactory'.

d) Let your educational supervisor know that the incoming DFT has a bad attitude.

e) Indicate your concerns on the feedback form with specific examples.

f) Give the student an opportunity to discuss the feedback with you and your educational supervisor.

g) Do not do anything as it is now too late for changes to be made.

h) Speak to your colleagues for advice.

30 Since your CQC inspection last year, standards seem to have slipped. Your dental chair has broken several times and the other day you discovered that you had no latex free gloves in the entire practice. What should you do?

Choose the three most appropriate answers when all of the answers are considered together.

a) Whinge to your fellow associates and patients.

b) Fix the chair yourself and buy your own gloves.

c) Report your concerns to the named person responsible.

d) Keep a written record of your concerns and any steps that you have taken.

e) Report your concerns at a practice meeting.

f) Report your concerns to the GDC.

g) Explain to the patients about your concerns.

h) Tell your practice manager that you will resign if nothing is done.

31 You arrive at work one morning and find one of your nurses shouting at an elderly patient. The tone and language are unpleasant. You know that the patient has early stages of dementia. What do you do?

Choose the three most appropriate answers when all of the answers are considered together.

a) Speak to the nurse immediately and stop the situation.

b) Discuss the situation with the practice manager.

c) Make preliminary enquiries from other staff to ask if they have seen similar behaviour.

d) Use body language to show your disapproval but do nothing formally.

e) Contact the GDC anonymously to avoid rousing the issue with your employers.

f) Do nothing for now.

g) Advise the nurse to leave the premises and not to return.

h) Seek advice from your indemnity provider.

32 You attend your induction for your new DFT job and are asked to sign an agreement never to raise concerns with bodies outside of your employing organization.

Choose the three most appropriate answers when all of the answers are considered together.

a) Sign and begin work as the practice is close to your home and it would be onerous to change.

b) Don't sign and hope that no one notices that it was not returned.

c) Explain that you cannot sign as it prohibits you from raising concerns appropriately about patient welfare.

d) Sign the form but resolve to raise concerns about patient safety in whatever way is needed.

e) Contact your indemnity provider.

f) Speak to senior colleagues for guidance and advice.

g) Contact the GDC.

h) Ask your DFT colleagues what they would do.

33 You are required to attend a postgraduate study day on a Friday as part of your DFT course. Your educational supervisor has asked you to work this coming Friday as he is short staffed.

Choose the three most appropriate answers when all of the answers are considered together.

a) Explain that the postgraduate day is mandatory and you are required to attend.

b) Get a friend to sign the attendance register and work on the day.

c) Agree that the practice comes first and stay.

d) Speak to your postgraduate educational supervisor for advice and guidance.

e) Make sure that reception blocks off your appointment book and clearly marks that it is a postgraduate study day.

f) Discuss with your other postgraduate colleagues.

g) Call your indemnity for advice.

h) Tell your educational supervisor that he is breaking the law.

34 A 30-year-old female attends your surgery. She has injuries to her teeth and jaws and lacerations to her face. She discloses that her partner has assaulted her and is very tearful. What do you do?

Choose the three most appropriate answers when all of the answers are considered together.

a) Attend to her dental injuries and tell her to go to accident and emergency.

b) Attend to her dental injuries, take photographs and document everything in detail.

c) Call social services.

d) Call the partner and tell him what you think of him!

e) Discuss your findings with the dedicated team lead for safeguarding adults in your practice.

f) Call for an ambulance so that her nondental injuries can be attended to.

g) Attend to her dental needs but do nothing more.

h) Attend to her dental needs and let her go, knowing that she will return again with the same old story.

35 Your patient experiences a vaso vagal attack in the chair. You ask your nurse for a glucose drink but she looks at you blankly and says that she does not know where the glucose is kept. What do you do?

Choose the three most appropriate answers when all of the answers are considered together.

a) Tell her and ask her to remember next time.

b) Tell her to get another colleague to assist.

c) Tell her where the glucose is kept and then speak to the practice manager about staff training.

d) Don't bother as the patient is feeling better.

e) Ask the nurse why she does not know once the patient has left.

f) Get angry.

g) Ask the practice manager to replace the nurse.

h) Give the patient your fizzy drink that you were saving for lunch.

36 You notice that one of the junior receptionists is eating lunch at her desk, always manning the phones until late and doing the early morning shift, opening up the surgery. There are other reception staff members that do not do all the extra shifts. You feel they are ganging up on the junior and making her always do the extra shifts. What do you do?

Choose the three most appropriate answers when all of the answers are considered together.

a) Call a staff meeting and bring up the issues so that everyone knows who the culprits are.

b) Speak to the practice manager about your findings and ask her to investigate further.

c) Call your indemnity provider for advice.

d) Speak to the junior receptionist and ask her to keep a log book, which you will show to the practice principal.

e) Speak to the other reception staff and accuse them of bullying the junior.

f) Don't get involved – they can organize their own rota themselves.

g) Sit both parties down with the practice manager and come to a solution that does not overwork any one person.

h) Tell your educational supervisor you think this is very rude and unfair.

37 Your nurse has mentioned that this is the third time in a week you have had emergency patients complaining that your filling left a large overhang that you must correct. She is concerned there is a pattern and wants you to bring this up with your educational supervisor. What do you do?

Choose the three most appropriate answers when all of the answers are considered together.

a) Ignore her, she is a nurse and does not know any better.

b) Agree politely but just monitor your work on your own instead.

c) Keep a log book and audit your work over the next few weeks, showing your educational supervisor your findings.

d) Reflect on what the nurse has stated in ePDP, showing this to your educational supervisor.

e) Speak to the practice manager, asking her to speak to your nurse about speaking out of turn.

f) Speak to the three patients and ask for their opinion.

g) Speak to the other associates and ask how they would handle the situation.

h) Go to your TPD about how you to deal with situations like these.

38 One of the head associates has taken the week off for a CPD training course abroad. You see on Facebook that he is uploading photos of himself relaxing by the pool and doing water sports. What do you do?

Choose the three most appropriate answers when all of the answers are considered together.

a) Tell the practice principal. You are annoyed as you have to see all his emergency patients.

b) Send him a quick message warning him about social media.

c) Show the pictures to the practice manager and tell her she can do what she pleases with the information.

d) Call the associate, telling him of your concern and ask him to please come clean on his return.

e) Call your indemnity provider for advice.

f) Don't say anything and pretend you haven't seen the photos.

g) Speak to the associate on their return at a practice meeting highlighting the issues involved.

h) Post a message on Facebook so that patients are aware of where he has gone.

39 You are extracting an upper left first molar when the root breaks. You continue to try removing the root tip when it propels into the maxillary sinus. You take radiographs to confirm that the root is sitting the lower portion of the antrum. What do you do?

Choose the three most appropriate answers when all of the answers are considered together.

a) The patient needs an explanation of what has happened.

b) Make a secondary referral.

c) Leave the root tip – it will hopefully be dormant.

d) Don't tell your patient anything for now.

e) Fill out an incident report form.

f) Make contemporaneous notes.

g) Tell the patient to take painkillers.

h) Give the patient antibiotics.

40 You are extracting a lower first molar. The procedure goes well and you send the patient away with all relevant postoperative instructions. After several hours your patient returns saying that his lip is still very numb; his lip and eyes seem droopy and he has noticed that his skin around his jaw is very pale. You suspect a facial palsy. What do you do?

Choose the three most appropriate answers when all of the answers are considered together.

a) Call your educational supervisor to go through the steps to take next.

b) Sympathize with the patient and explain what has occurred.

c) Call your indemnity provider for advice.

d) Ask for further educational supervisor tutorials to be focused around local anaesthesia.

e) Carry out a full investigation. Refer the patient and review in 2 weeks.

f) Ask for this patient to be seen by oral medicine and make a referral as appropriate.

g) Tell the patient not to worry and that everything will be alright.

h) Tell him to go home and carry on as normal.

41 You are reading through the staff certificates, registrations and CPD when you see that one of the longstanding associates has had CPD every year for medical emergencies; however, no one in the practice recalls ever seeing him attend a medical emergency session. This associate is not a member of any other practice and seems to have had the time and date signed off even though he was not in attendance. What do you do?

Choose the three most appropriate answers when all of the answers are considered together.

a) Pretend you have not noticed this in the folder.

b) Highlight this to the practice manager, advising her to take this further.

c) Bring this up at a practice meeting, highlighting your concerns for CPD.

d) Do an audit on CPD in the practice and present your results at a practice meeting.

e) Speak to the associate with your educational supervisor, advising him to speak to his indemnity provider.

f) Report him to the GDC.

g) Discuss the situation with your colleagues immediately.

h) Advise him to start documenting his CPD correctly.

42 You are taking routine bitewings for a regular patient who has been coming to see you during your DF1 year. You see some interproximal radiolucency suggesting caries. On probing, the surface seems roughened but firm, hard

and scratchy. Explaining the carious lesion as mild but present to the patient you both decide to leave the tooth and use fluoride application, good cleaning and regular visits to the dentist. Six months later there is a short, sharp pain from the tooth and the patient attends with a written complaint to the practice against you for this occurring. What do you do?

Choose the three most appropriate answers when all of the answers are considered together.

a) Seek advice from your educational supervisor and TPD immediately.

b) Call your indemnity provider for advice.

c) Ask the patient to attend a meeting with you, your educational supervisor and practice manager to discuss the patient's concern.

d) Offer the patient a free hygiene visit for their inconvenience after you have treated their pain.

e) Document all aspects of the complaint and write up a full log in the incident report form using this as a basis for an audit and peer review.

f) Apologize to the patient and say that it is not your responsibility that this has happened.

g) Offer to take more routine radiographs.

h) Offer the patient a settlement for him to drop the complaint.

43 You just complete a long RCT treatment on a patient with a clear medical history when your receptionist asks you to take a call outside from the local lab. You instruct the nurse to sit the patient back up and provide her with a rinse. On returning you find the patient lying on the floor and your nurse looking extremely distressed. She informs you that the patient stood up, felt dizzy and fainted, falling to the floor. You ask her to get the oxygen but it becomes clear that your nurse has no idea what to do or how to act in this medical emergency. What do you do?

Choose the three most appropriate answers when all of the answers are considered together.

a) Call 999.

b) Ask her to call for help and find someone who can bring the oxygen and medical emergency kit.

c) At a practice meeting, bring up your concern about medical emergencies and suggest further training be given to all staff.

d) Train your nurse in basic resuscitation but suggest that she seek further training.

e) Make the practice principal fully aware of the situation.

f) Attend to the patient, carrying out basic life support until the patient has regained consciousness.

g) Do nothing as you assume that the patient will regain consciousness soon.

h) Report her to the GDC as you feel she is not competent.

44 A non-English-speaking patient whose language you speak discloses that she lives with a family as a domestic worker. She is never allowed to leave alone and given very little money. She is made to work long hours and is not allowed a mobile phone. She is very unhappy but does the work as she can send money back home to her impoverished family. You feel very uncomfortable about this situation. What do you do?

Choose the three most appropriate answers when all of the answers are considered together.

a) Do nothing as it is none of your business.

b) Speak to your TPD as you know that he is caring and will make a decision for you.

c) Speak to your educational supervisor as you are concerned for this vulnerable adult.

d) Call your indemnity provider with a view to calling social services.

e) Try to forget this experience.

f) Write good, contemporaneous notes.

g) Ask another colleague to see the patient next time.

h) Accept the situation as a cultural view.

45 Your patient has a very extensive medical history, a lot of which involves medicines you have not heard of and do not know the mechanisms of. You are worried about beginning treatment in this position. What do you do?

Choose the three most appropriate answers when all of the answers are considered together.

a) Stop treatment to look up the medicines in the BNF before you commence.

b) Speak to your educational supervisor for extra medical history and drug tutorials.

c) Continue with treatment as the patient informs you these medicines don't interact with any form of dental treatment.

d) Make contemporaneous notes, outlining that you did not know the drug mechanisms.

e) Ask for a second opinion from one of the associates before beginning treatment.

f) Before the full examination, research all the drugs and their mechanisms, especially any side effects and dental-related interactions.

g) Carry on, as most medicines do not really interfere with dental treatment.

h) Use a very old BNF to find out more about the drugs.

46 You feel that your educational supervisor picks on you in front of all the nurses to make himself look better. You are finding it increasingly hard to sit in at lunch or practice meetings. One on one he is fine and actually a very good educational supervisor; however his humiliating you in public is affecting your confidence. What do you do?

Choose the three most appropriate answers when all of the answers are considered together.

a) Express your feelings to your practice manager, seeking her advice.
b) Speak to your TPD about your feelings and ask for advice on how to move forward.
c) Ask to be moved to a different training practice as your morale is very low.
d) Approach your educational supervisor to discuss your feelings to see whether you can work something out together.
e) Avoid public areas and be quiet in practice meetings.
f) Ask the other associates if they are having a similar experience; if so, then you know it is not personal at least.
g) Call in sick.
h) Try to toughen up so that you can brush off these comments.

47 There is a big commotion in the waiting room. You are in-between patients so you go out to see what is going on. You see a mother punching her child in the face. The children have always been very quiet, introverted and the mother obnoxious and rude. You have noticed that the child has bruises across his neck. What do you do?

Choose the three most appropriate answers when all of the answers are considered together.

a) Call social services to explain your concerns regarding this family.
b) Write a full record of the event in an incidence report form, which you need to show to the practice principal as soon as possible.
c) Do not panic. Involve the wider team in the scenario so that you can all help to control this situation.
d) Ignore the commotion and return to writing up your notes.
e) Call the practice principal to attend to the child immediately.
f) Call your indemnity for impartial advice.
g) Let someone else deal with the problem.
h) Ignore, as the mother is allowed to discipline her child.

48 You are working on a patient when the bur falls out of the hand piece and down the patient's throat. What do you do?

Choose the three most appropriate answers when all of the answers are considered together.

a) Stop treatment, stabilizing the patient and send him for a chest x-ray.
b) Ask your nurse to put the suction down the throat to see if she can retrieve the bur.
c) Stop treatment and explain what has occurred to the patient and, if he is happy, then carry on treatment.
d) Call your educational supervisor in for advice on how to proceed in this situation.
e) Write contemporaneous notes on the appointment.

f) Write up an incidence report form giving a copy to the practice manager.

g) Do not say anything, as you are confident that the bur will pass through the digestive system.

h) Tell the patient not to worry as everything will be alright.

49 One of your patients discloses that he has a severe drug addiction problem and has also been thinking of self-harming. What do you do?

Choose the three most appropriate answers when all of the answers are considered together.

a) Increase the patient recall time to ensure that regular maintenance occurs.

b) Monitor the problem and, when appropriate, refer to the patient's GP for medical attention.

c) Call the police, as your patient is in possession of class A drugs.

d) Call the patient's GP immediately, informing him of your findings, taking a multidisciplinary approach.

e) Give drug-cessation advice to the patient – advising him to seek further help.

f) Let him carry on as he is – it is his life after all.

g) Do nothing as you cannot be bothered with patients like this.

h) Tell him that he is wasting his life and to stop taking drugs immediately.

50 A patient complains to the reception that his wallet went missing from his coat while he went in for treatment. What do you do?

Choose the three most appropriate answers when all of the answers are considered together.

a) Apologize to the patient.

b) Ensure that a thorough investigation will be held.

c) Keep the patient informed of any conclusions.

d) Ask the reception staff to tell you who they suspect most.

e) Take some petty cash to reimburse the patient.

f) Ask the patient if he is sure that he had his wallet with him.

g) Ask your nurse if she knows who took the wallet.

h) Tell the patient that he is responsible for his own belongings.

51 There are a lot of patients who cannot read English within the practice and have asked for signs to be in Arabic. What do you do?

Choose the three most appropriate answers when all of the answers are considered together.

a) Do a survey for all patients to see if the majority would like this implementation.

b) Refuse as English is the primary language in the United Kingdom.

c) All signs should be changed from English to Arabic immediately.

d) Ask these patient to seek dentistry elsewhere.

e) Come up with a plan for important signs to be translated and discuss this at a practice meeting.
f) Identify other problems that these patients may experience during their visits.
g) Put up a notice advertising a local English-language school.
h) Refuse as this would cost far too much.

52 You note there is no disabled ramp in the entrance of the practice. You bring this up at a staff meeting where the practice manager says there is no need as there are no disabled patents at this practice. What do you do?

Choose the three most appropriate answers when all of the answers are considered together.
a) Speak to your practice principal about the legality behind this issue.
b) Call your indemnity provider regarding what should be done.
c) Call the builder and pay for the installation of a ramp yourself.
d) Call a meeting with the practice principal and practice manager highlighting the importance of the ramp.
e) Take the practice manager's point as valid.
f) Only accept patients that are mobile and do not require this facility.
g) Ask patients to bring their own ramp with them for dental appointments.
h) Do nothing as all your parents are able bodied.

53 You have had a busy, stressful morning with difficult, long treatments. You have been asked to see an emergency patient just before lunch. The patient requires an extraction of the LL6, which is causing him pain. You are about to start the extraction when the patient asks you why you gave him the injection on the right side?

Choose the three most appropriate answers when all of the answers are considered together.
a) Apologize for your mistake.
b) Call your educational supervisor for advice. You are clearly very tired and need assistance.
c) Numb the other side of the mouth too and continue with the treatment.
d) Speak to your educational supervisor after asking if patients cannot be squeezed into your diary without asking you.
e) Rebook the patient for another day as you cannot numb both sides.
f) Call in sick the next day and take a long vacation.
g) Discuss work/life balance with your colleagues.
h) Become irritated with yourself as you know that you have made a mistake.

54 Your patient begins to breathe heavily and complains of a pain from his chest. He has previously had a heart attack. You can see the patient is becoming more breathless. You see from his medical history the patient has high blood pressure and that he has been taking statins for his cholesterol.

Choose the three most appropriate answers when all of the answers are considered together.
a) Ask your nurse to get the first-aid trolley.
b) Call for help and an ambulance as soon as possible.
c) Give GTN sublingually.
d) Reassure the patient and do nothing more.
e) Ask your nurse to turn the air conditioning up.
f) Sit the patient up.
g) Lie the patient down.
h) Quickly finish the dental treatment.

55 A mother and her child attend your surgery for their dental health assessment. You assess the mother first whilst her son sits on the extra chair in your surgery. At first glance the child looks unkempt, with torn clothes, various scratch marks and frightened. You go through the mother's medical history and notice that she is a heroin user and is currently taking methadone to help her addiction. After completing the mother's assessment, she goes to stand next to the door to make a phone call. When assessing the child you immediately notice rampant caries and the child informs you his mum often gives him sweet strawberry medicine to help him sleep more.

Choose the three most appropriate answers when all of the answers are considered together.
a) Complete your contemporaneous notes at the end of the appointment and take the case to the child protection lead in the practice with a view to taking this further.
b) Report the mother to social services as you suspect child neglect.
c) Call your educational supervisor in for advice.
d) Speak to your indemnity provider for impartial advice.
e) Ignore the unkempt signs as you can't be entirely sure and deal with the dental issues only.
f) Accuse the mother of drugging her child and causing dental and general neglect.
g) Confront the mother directly, as you are angry.
h) Call 999.

56 You notice that your educational supervisor has been referring all his extractions either to hospital, a specialist practice in the local area or rebooking the patients with another practitioner in the practice. You've also noticed that whenever you need help with an extraction he is always conveniently busy or refuses to help you with the treatment. You feel this issue needs to be raised. What do you do?

Choose the three most appropriate answers when all of the answers are considered together.
a) Speak to other associates and see if they have noticed the issue too.

b) Speak to your TPD in regards to the issue, showing them a log book of events.

c) Confront your educational supervisor on an occasion when he refuses to perform an extraction, persuading him to seek help.

d) Suggest at a practice meeting all associates go on extra CPD with oral surgery.

e) Bring up what you have discovered with your educational supervisor, practice principal and another associate, trying to help him become more confident in oral surgery.

f) Raise this concern with the GDC.

g) Offer to do the extractions yourself.

h) Do nothing as it is none of your business.

57 After a few months you receive your first complaint from a woman who did not receive her treatment plan in writing as promised. There was a series of events that led to the complaint but ultimately the blame lies with you as the dental practitioner. You call the woman to apologize and reassure her that the letter has been sent by first class. The patient still wants to put this complaint forward. What do you do?

Choose the three most appropriate answers when all of the answers are considered together.

a) There is no need for your educational supervisors or practice manager to know that the practice received a complaint.

b) Make contemporaneous notes, explain what occurred at a practice meeting and come up with ideas to ensure complaints are minimized.

c) Write up the complaint alone and add it to the complaint folder.

d) Tell the practice manager about the complaint and suggest that you will audit complaints.

e) Ask your educational supervisor if the next tutorial can be based around complaint handling.

f) Transfer the patient to another associate's list to ensure you do not have to handle her again.

g) Do nothing and hope the patient forgets to act upon her complaint.

h) Tell her to calm down, hoping she will drop the written complaint claims.

58 Your practice is piloting a new composite resin material and is heavily endorsing the product. At a practice meeting the manager states that all associates need to use the material when placing white fillings. It is a very new product with which you are unfamiliar. What do you do?

Choose the three most appropriate answers when all of the answers are considered together.

a) Agree with the manager and start endorsing the product too.

b) Ask your educational supervisor to shadow you the first few times you are using it, for guidance.

c) Try on a phantom head first and build up your confidence until you are happy.

d) Explain to the manager that you will use whichever resin material is in the best interest of the specific patient's case.

e) Refuse to endorse any product at all.

f) Discuss what to do with your flatmates.

g) Only use it on elderly patients.

h) Call the GDC for advice.

59 On your study day, your DF1 colleague confides in you that he is being investigated for a potential diagnosis of HIV. Your colleague is worried he might have contracted the virus and asks you for your advice. He would appreciate that you keep the matter confidential.

Choose the three most appropriate answers when all of the answers are considered together.

a) Report your colleague to the GDC.

b) Advise your colleague to make an appointment with occupational health to get a checkup.

c) Advise your colleague to contact his indemnity.

d) Advise your colleague to speak to his educational supervisor.

e) Advise your colleague that regulations have changed and dentists with HIV can still legally work so just book an appointment with his GP to get checked.

f) Advise your colleague not to worry as the changes of transmission are low and he would have known by now if he had the virus.

g) Advise you colleague to cancel all his patients and take sick leave until he has had a checkup from occupational health.

h) Seek advice from your indemnity provider.

60 The principal dentist in your practice has called in sick. Your practice manager has allocated his patients between you and the other two associate dentists. You treat Mr Smith with a continued root-canal treatment on a lower right 6. The principal dentist had extirpated and prepared the distal canal in Mr Smith's appointment last week. You numb the patient and go on to place the rubber dam. The patient seems confused and asks you what the rubber dam is used for. After explaining the importance of the rubber dam to the patient, Mr Smith informs you that the principal dentist didn't use one last time. The patient seems quite annoyed and continues to say he feels the principal dentist is always trying to take short cuts and does not do things properly. How do you respond to the patient's accusations?

Choose the three most appropriate answers when all of the answers are considered together.

a) Reassure the patient for now, stating you will look into the matter further once the principal dentist is back at work.

b) Agree with the patient, encouraging him to make a formal complaint about this malpractice.

c) Ask your nurse to compare with the patient the two root-canal appointments as she was present for both.

d) Listen to the patient's grievances; ask if he would like this matter to be taken further and call the patient for a review.

e) Ignore the patient's comments and continue with the treatment.

f) Tell the patient the principal will never listen to you as you are only a foundation dentist.

g) Write up the patient's words in your notes after completing the root-canal treatment.

h) Assure the patient that the procedure will be a 100% success.

61 You attend your practice to realize that you are the only dentist on site. There are no nurses either and only one receptionist, who is not GDC registered.

Choose the three most appropriate answers when all of the answers are considered together.

a) Ask the practice manager to arrange for a locum nurse immediately.

b) Cancel all patients as soon as possible.

c) Prioritize those patients who may have pain or be in emergency need.

d) Call your educational supervisor, asking him to come in and help sort out this situation.

e) Refuse to treat any patients at all and leave.

f) Report the practice to the CQC.

g) Make a reflection log on your EPDP.

h) Close the practice so no patients can come in.

62 A patient sees you for emergency treatment. He reports that he had two molar teeth out 3 days ago in this practice and is in great pain. He feels that he has been 'butchered' by your associate and wants to know from you if there is enough evidence to sue the other dentist.

Choose the three most appropriate answers when all of the answers are considered together.

a) Deal with the dental problems and say nothing.

b) Explain that he should sue as you have heard that there have been problems with that dentist before.

c) Deal with his pain, reassure the patient and ask him to come back in a few days to discuss the matter further when he is not suffering pain.

d) Phone your defence union.

e) Inform the treating dentist what has occurred, asking him to speak to the patient directly.

f) Tell the patient to stop exaggerating; postoperative pain is common after an extraction.

g) Blame the patient and say it's because of him smoking and not following postoperative instructions correctly.

h) Review the patient in 6 months' time.

63 A noncooperative and rude patient tells you that he does not wish to reveal his medical history and just wants you to get on with things as he is in pain.

Choose the three most appropriate answers when all of the answers are considered together.

a) Tell him to go somewhere else as you are busy today.

b) Advise him that without the medical history there will only be a limited number of treatments that you will be able to do for him.

c) Advise him that, for his own safety, you need full details of his medical history.

d) Tell him that he is being very irresponsible.

e) Treat him anyway as you have a duty of care to patients in care.

f) Ask a more senior colleague to come in and reinforce the advice you gave to the patient as this may help.

g) Ask a colleague to see him.

h) Tell him that you cannot help him under the current circumstances as it is not in his best interest.

64 A senior associate is away on holiday. Your educational supervisor and you are seeing the associate's patients whilst they are away as a goodwill gesture. You go to fit a crown when the patient presents with gross caries on the prep. The crown fits well.

Choose the three most appropriate answers when all of the answers are considered together.

a) Fit the crown and recall as necessary.

b) Explain that there is caries on the prep.

c) Do not fit the crown and rearrange an appointment with the associate.

d) Call your educational supervisor in to look at the tooth.

e) Write contemporaneous notes.

f) Highlight this issue at the next practice meeting.

g) Tell the patient your findings of caries and what your professional opinion is in future treatment.

h) Speak to the associate on their return regarding this patient with your educational supervisor present.

65 You are in a dual foundation-year practice so there are two foundation dentists (FD) and two foundation educational supervisors. You notice that the other FD and his educational supervisor have a very good relationship and he is progressing much quicker than you are. You are finding it difficult to sync with your educational supervisor and generally finding the FD process very slow and no progression being made.

Choose the three most appropriate answers when all of the answers are considered together.

a) Speak to the other FD in the practice to speak to their educational supervisor to help.

b) Speak to your TPD for advice.

c) Call the GDC.

d) Ask the practice manager to organize more team-building skill days.

e) Continue with the FD experience as you don't want to be seen as a complainer.

f) Speak to the FDs on your scheme complaining that the other FD keeps showing off.

g) Explain your situation to your undergraduate tutor.

h) Ask your nurse to tell your educational supervisor about how you are feeling.

66 You look ahead in your diary to the following week and notice that you have a study day scheduled and the reception staff have booked in a full day of patients in error on the same day. Study days are mandatory but you do not want to cause issues at your practice either.

Choose the three most appropriate answers when all of the answers are considered together.

a) Inform your TPD about what has occurred so that all parties are aware and have enough notice to resolve the situation.

b) Speak to your educational supervisors and explain the error that has been made.

c) Call your patients yourself and explain that you are an FD and this is mandatory.

d) Call the practice principal, complaining about the inconvenience this has caused you.

e) Try to work with the rest of the team in correcting this diary mistake.

f) Make a complaint to the practice manager about the reception staff as they should know better since they have a list of all your study-day dates.

g) Call your indemnity provider.

h) Ignore the error and plan to call in sick to your study day so no one is inconvenienced.

67 You are seeing a family of patients at the end of your day. You notice:

° you only have 5 minutes per child and 20 minutes for the mother;

° there are seven children attending today;

° children range in age from 3 years to 17 years;

° these are new patients.

Choose the three most appropriate answers when all of the answers are considered together.

a) Forewarn your educational supervisor of the situation so she is aware to be around if help is needed.

b) Ask your educational supervisor and other dentists in the practice if they are able to fit in a few of the older children.

c) Speak about the incident at a practice meeting/tutorial and come up with a suitable plan to time manage well in situations like this.

d) Refuse to see the family as the appointment duration is out of your remit. Ask reception to rearrange their appointments more suitably.

e) Tell the mother that this is unacceptable and to consider her parenting skills.

f) Tell reception to rearrange the older children's appointments as you refuse to see them in such a short appointment time.

g) Report the whole incident to your TPD.

h) See all the patients, doesn't matter if you know you are going to overrun. It's not your fault they were all booked for the end of the day.

68 Your nurse and the receptionist do not get along. At first you found your nurse complaining amusing; however, now your nurse always seems distressed after dealing with reception and you have caught your nurse crying in the staff room. What do you do?

Choose the three most appropriate answers when all of the answers are considered together.

a) Ask the practice manager to speak to both parties seeking a resolution.

b) Comfort your nurse but urge her to speak out about how she is feeling.

c) Speak to the principal, asking her to bring up the importance of working as a team and respecting one another at the next practice meeting.

d) Log all activity you notice to assess the severity of the issue.

e) Ignore the situation as it will eventually resolve.

f) Keep an eye on the reception staff and note the first time they make any mistake.

g) Ask your TPD to change your practice as you are finding the politics distracting.

h) Tell your nurse that these situations occur regularly in working practice. She needs to not let them affect her and to be stronger.

69 You are seeing a child for an initial examination. When you write up the treatment plan, the parents disagree with majority of what is outlined and demand alternatives. The majority of alternatives for the teeth in question are to do nothing which will undoubtedly will cause pain, swelling or issues in the future for this child.

Choose the three most appropriate answers when all of the answers are considered together.

a) Speak to your educational supervisor privately in regards to this case asking for detailed advice.

b) Allow the parents to vent but continue with the treatment plan you have written up.

c) Dismiss the parents' concerns and write up your notes on your clinical examination.

d) Note all conversations down in contemporaneous note form.

e) Explain all outcomes and options to the parents giving your professional opinion on the matter.

f) Speak to social services about your concerns on these parents.

g) Brush the patient's teeth and send the family on their way.

h) Agree with whatever plan the patient's parents put together.

70 A patient attends with a cold sore. It is practice policy not to see any patients with cold sores. The patient has waited for this appointment for nearly a month. What do you do?

Choose the three most appropriate answers when all of the answers are considered together.

a) Explain the practice policy to the patient and empathize with the patient's inconvenience.

b) Ask your educational supervisor if you can take a quick look.

c) Advise the patient to purchase OTC acyclovir and analgesics if necessary.

d) Bring this scenario up in a practice meeting and ask other clinicians on their views.

e) Treat the patient as normal as it is unethical to let them leave untreated.

f) Ask the patient to leave and stop being so inconsiderate.

g) Call the reception staff, telling them off for even allowing the patient into the surgery.

h) Rebook the patient in next week when the cold sore should have healed.

71 A patient attends for an extirpation of his UL2. On attendance, the patient strongly smells of marijuana and seems absent. When explaining the extirpation treatment the patient seems distant and agrees with all you are saying. You feel uncomfortable treating the patient today. What would you do?

Choose the three most appropriate answers when all of the answers are considered together.

a) Carry on with the extirpation. You are running late as it is and it is in the patient's best interest.

b) The patient consented for treatment at his examination appointment so it does not really matter if he is under the influence of drugs or not.

c) Instant message your educational supervisor asking her to discretely assist you in obtaining a valid medical history and consent.

d) Alongside your nurse, note down how the patient is reacting and make sure that you are not making an assumption.

e) Ask the patient for an up-to-date medical history ensuring that you ask if he uses recreational drugs.

f) Write all conversations down in contemporaneous notes.

g) Disregard your suspicions as it is rude and judgemental.

h) Confront the patient and ask him to rebook when he is more focused.

72 A patient is complaining loudly at the reception desk as you are calling your patient in. The receptionist is on her own and seems scared. What do you do?

Choose the three most appropriate answers when all of the answers are considered together.

a) Ask your patient to wait in your surgery whilst you help the reception deal with this patient.

b) Try to move the patient to a side room to discuss the matters further.

c) Call the practice principal immediately to address the complaint whilst you attend to your patient.

d) Ignore the situation and continue with your patient.

e) Take your patient in and ask your nurse to deal with the commotion outside.

f) Hand gesture to the receptionist, advising her to hurry up in calming the patient down.

g) Ask your patient to sort out this fiasco by explaining what a lovely experience she is having.

h) Ignore your patient and help your receptionist deal with the angry patient.

73 You are constantly late to work as you live so far away, you are finding the commute difficult and do not want to make a bad impression on the practice owners or educational supervisors. One day you are nearly an hour late and patients have to be rescheduled. Your educational supervisor does not say much except how this is becoming too much of a habit. You are feeling upset with this comment. What do you do?

Choose the three most appropriate answers when all of the answers are considered together.

a) Explain your predicament to the educational supervisor and practice principal trying to put a more appropriate plan in place.

b) Apologize for your lateness but fully explain your circumstances.

c) Ignore the educational supervisor's comments as you cannot control traffic in the mornings.

d) Speak to your educational supervisor on their comment explaining how you felt uncomfortable and upset.

e) Try to stay away from your educational supervisor for the rest of the day.

f) Speak to your TPD in regards to the whole scenario to help advise further.

g) Quit the FD programme as you are too tired to continue.

h) Ask the reception team to book in a 'fake' patient in your 9 a.m. slot, so even if you do run late no patients are affected.

74 The nurses have a private 'whatsapp' group where they discuss the daily activities in the practice in a mocking manner. They have added you to this group as they feel that, as a younger member of the team, you would appreciate their comments. You notice some of the comments are crude, unprofessional and, if ever any of the messages were leaked, would shed a bad light on your practice and have serious consequences on the members in the group. What do you do?

Choose the three most appropriate answers when all of the answers are considered together.

a) Leave the group.

b) Explain to the nursing staff how unprofessional and dangerous the group is.

c) Report the group to the GDC.

d) Strongly advise nurses to complain in a professional manner.

e) The group is private so there is no problem in being involved.

f) Stay in the group but do not comment.

g) Copy the group conversation for the entire practice to read.

h) Participate in the group as you feel accepted by the nursing team and have your own frustrations to vent.

75 You are completing a CQC outcome report for your practice when you realize that the compliance for less-abled people such as ramps into the practice and disabled toilets is poor. There is no CQC lead for 'access' to the practice and the last audit done on access was over ten years ago. When you ask the practice manager why there is no disabled access or focus on this she says the owner's ethos is not to treat disabled people. What do you do?

Choose the three most appropriate answers when all of the answers are considered together.

a) Call CQC and ask them to intervene.

b) Call the GDC and ask them to intervene.

c) Speak to your TPD for their advice.

d) Speak to an associate for advice.

e) Speak to your educational supervisor for advice.

f) Call the police.

g) Accept the situation and carry on as normal. It is not your responsibility.

h) Ask your fellow FDs in your scheme if their practices have similar issues.

'Best-of-three' SJTs: Answers

Answers are from the GDC, used with permission. Information is correct at the time of going to press. Please visit the GDC web site to check for any changes since publication: www.gdc-uk.org (accessed 10 November 2015).

1 CDF

Asking the patient for a history of the incident, so that you can take this forward, shows logical reasoning. It also ensures that you are putting the patient's complaint first. This, and involving the wider team by sending an email to all colleagues and notifying the local authority, is the best combination. You would not imply the patient is at fault as A and E suggested, nor should you without evidence accuse any staff members as B suggests.

2 DGH

Asking your educational supervisor first is the best plan, especially if you feel uncomfortable or if this is your first time handling trauma with children. G is obvious but in a stressful situation it may be difficult to act methodically and in a logical manner. Take great care in treating this patient sympathetically and ensuring all relevant preop and postop information is given to the patient. By questioning the teacher you gain a thorough history, document all this in notes and are in a stronger position if there are any future dento-legal concerns. DGH are a good combination as they handle all clinical and administrative issues and deal with all protocols in place for such incidents. A is negligent as you only have 15 minutes to act. C does not deal with the tooth problem and at present the patient will not need to visit Accident and Emergency, as she is only a little dizzy. Your postop instructions would have provided the patient on information about head injury. E is unnecessary as general dental practitioners should be competent to deal with such incidents and F is negligent. B is valid; however, G is more applicable in this instance.

3 BCH

BCH are the best suited together. Option B shows that you abide by the GDC standards and have taken your oath seriously – although this may be a very difficult scenario, especially is your educational supervisor is at fault here. H deals with what has been asked by you. Informing your educational supervisor about why you are refusing means that you have acted in good faith, informing him of what must be done. C is a good idea to save any dento-legal issues. Writing a log book of events with times/dates of conversations with any witnesses is a good idea as your indemnity provider can then follow a paper trail of events if necessary. A is illegal and D shows bad faith to the profession. F has no relevance to dentistry as the authorities to be visited would be the GDC. E and G are valid but not just yet. You could ask your scheme leader for advice but do not necessarily report your educational supervisor yet unless he does not rectify his mistakes. It is again a little too early to inform the patient, as E suggests, as your educational supervisor may do this himself or herself. Always give the team a chance to act lawfully and rectify mistakes before acting yourself.

4 AEF

It is not your responsibility, under the Employment Act, to deal with this scenario. A and F are very justifiable, as other members of the team have this responsibility, especially as a foundation dentist you do not have any educational supervisor in team management and handling. Out of all the options left, E is what you would do as a professional, as B and H do not handle the situation head on but are a coward's way out; C and D are unprofessional and will embarrass the nurse and G is very blunt and could be deemed as rude.

5 ACD

You need immediate help from senior members of staff – A and C are good together as they include the wider team and also tackle future learning and reflection from this issue. D ensures the safety of your patient and that he is informed of the delay for now. B, E, F and G are all very extreme. H is unprofessional and illegal.

6 ACE

C is first. Asking your educational supervisor once a full history and examination has been completed will aid you in further treatment and your educational supervisor can help you formulate a plan. Asking your educational supervisor also gives you confidence to treat the child as two dental practitioners would have reviewed the patient's case. A shows initiative, especially if the child is in pain and is of Gillick competence. A follow up shows care and respect for protocol too. E allows the parents to be fully informed so they are aware of the appointment and treatment – ideally a courtesy call could be made just before treatment and a message left, at least. B is not active and is something that should have been done before starting at the practice in induction. D is valid; however, it is unnecessary, especially if you have your educational supervisor to seek advice from first. F could be deemed negligent, especially if the child goes and gains a large facial swelling, pyrexia, or cyst-like features. G is polite; however, you could tell the patients this once they are in your surgery room. H is unprofessional – it is not acting in the best interest of the patient nor is it acting as a good team member.

7 DEG

All issues should be handled in house first ideally, so H and C are unnecessary at present. B and G are similar; however, G has more team members involved and so has your TPD, who can handle the whole situation better. D is definitely valid and should be done as soon as you realize the extent of the situation. E is more useful than F, especially as this is induction and a staff meeting may be daunting. There may be wider issues to deal with than an indemnity provider can advise on. Staff meetings are more for when are you a part of the team. This questions implies that this is your first week of induction and this is a 'raising concerns' issue.

8 ADF

D is the best option. Start by organizing yourself. Make a plan and reassure yourself that you can redeem yourself. Once you have showed this to your educational supervisor you can move forward on how to rectify the mistake you have made. F allows you to gain support from your TPD as this is the person who will also be signing off ePDP alongside your educational supervisor. The TPD's input is as valued as your educational supervisor's here. Showing that you have made a plan also demonstrates initiative. Speaking to your educational supervisor, as A states, now puts a plan into place and includes the wider team. All other options do not handle the problem at hand with the appropriate members.

9 ACD

C must be done first. Deal with the nurse confiding in you and tell her the relevant documents from which she should seek guidance. A can be done as a paper trail so that the practice principal can look into the matter and train the nurse appropriately. D deals with the actual issue involved – CPD training. It also involves the practice manager, who can look into this whole issue, including any CQC issues involving infection control. B is out of your remit as a foundation dentist. The training should be left to the practice manager or principal. E is a suggestion rather providing information. F is negligent and H is extreme, especially if she is a trainee. G is valid; however, this is a future learning outcome for the greater team and yourself. Future audits could be carried out on infection control, too, in order to learn from this incident.

10 ABC

B, C and A are the best combination when considered together. A is administrative, B enables you to gain advice and C shows initiative in the future action plan. D and H are valid but try to handle this situation in house first. E is extreme. F is not logical as you cannot be expected to complete exams in 15 minutes with no prior experience in doing so with this time limit. G is unprofessional.

11 ADF

Always put the patients' best interests first and advise them professionally what you have investigated and concluded – this is the case in A. D and F are an excellent combination as your educational supervisor and wider team are involved plus the advice of your indemnity provider here can prove to help you follow the correct steps in ensuring patients' safety. B is negligent. C is too extreme at this stage. E is unnecessary considering that it is one associate's problem rather than a problem affecting the whole team. G and H are good but not relevant to the questions as yet.

12 BCF

BCF are a good combination. B deals directly with the source of the problem. C includes your educational supervisor in the scenario and F ensures that the team learns from the mistakes being made. D, G and H are all very extreme and E is passing the buck and not taking responsibility for what you have found out. A is not an option as it would be unprofessional to turn a blind eye.

13 BCG

As B suggests, dealing with a patient in a social environment is not professional and could undermine confidentiality, hence AEFH are not applicable. D, acting in compensation, is unethical and the GDC could regard it as trying to bribe the patient to deter him from taking this matter further. C needs to occur even if it is outside of the practice parameters and G gives a step-by-step account of how to act in this situation.

14 EFG

G comes first, as your educational supervisor will aid you in this matter. E is necessary as the patient-dentist relationship may be under scrutiny here and F will ensure that the associate is reminded of the rules and regulations regarding this relationship. A is the easy option but remember that you have a duty of care to all patients. B is extreme at this stage. C is very similar to E; however, he should not be left to disclose this at his own leisure. H is inappropriate.

15 ACE

A needs to be done quickly at the time of witnessing the act as all members of the team who are registered have a responsibility to act within their scope of practice. C is key, especially as CPD is a continuation and, if nurses are not up to date on this, incidents like these can occur. E must be done; it is important not only to educate other members of the team but to ensure that a written note of any events is logged at the time and date they occur. E ensures that the matter is handled locally first – as H suggests. GDC can be included at a later date if applicable. B and D are negligent. F and G are good options; however, C and E are better options.

16 DEH

D is the perfect answer here. Calling your patient in means that you can speak to him regarding diagnosis. Speaking to the receptionists will stop them from making diagnoses that could be detrimental to other patients in the waiting room. E and H are good follow-on points. E ensures that the wider team can learn and discuss the incidents. It gives an opportunity for reflection and, potentially, audit. H ensures that reception staff receive frequent and up-to-date training, as they are members of a professional team and need relevant training to ensure that this issue does not occur again. ABC are unprofessional. You should not divulge any information to the patient nor inform the staff members about issues in front of patients. G is extreme. F does not prove that you can act as a team player – by just handing in a form you are not actually dealing with the event that has occurred, nor are you moving forward by suggesting any training or time for reflection for the staff members involved.

17 ABG

Reassurance and communication are key, especially when managing patient expectations – A deals with these issues. Discussing options with your educational supervisor ensures that all advice given to the patient can be discussed between the three of you. It also allows your educational supervisor to help reassure the patients and their demands. This is an interesting case, so reflecting on how you could have handled the situation better – what you did well and what you did less well – would be very helpful in your further professional development. Hence G is a good option. C and H may be your professional opinion; however, this does not show good communication skills or an interest in what the patient's concern is. D and E use the word 'threat', which is not necessarily what the patient's mother's concern is. F is not applicable; this is not an incident – this is a regular primary concern.

18 ADF

A, D and F are the best options when considered together. A – deal with the patient in the chair, finish treatment and ensure safety for him. D – speak to your educational supervisor or TPD as soon as possible. F – if the complaint is serious and needs dento-legal advice, seek this as soon as possible. All other options here are not applicable, unprofessional or show negligence.

19 DFG

This is a medical emergency issue. DFG are what is stated in the resuscitation guidelines. F – calling for help, D – ensuring complete safety for the patient and administering the drugs, G – ensuring the future drug supply (in this case oxygen) is prepared. All other options are not in the guidelines, so a basic understanding of the steps taken to ensure patient safety in a medical emergency need to be considered and adapted to the scenario given. See the Resuscitation Council UK guidelines for more details.

20 BDF

This is not necessarily something that the educational supervisors, TPDs and the team need to be told about straight away. Firstly, it is better for your colleague to gain a better understanding of his medical conditions as B and F suggest. This is a sensitive topic and an indemnity provider would be able to give valid, impartial advice as D suggests whereas it might be difficult to speak to other members of the dental foundation scheme.

21 AEH

Scope of practice is not to be undermined and is taken very seriously by the GDC – ensure A is done tactfully but quickly. E is appropriate as well to ensure that the nurse takes what she is doing seriously. H ensures further professional development with radiology and scope of practice as potential subject titles. B is out of the nurse's scope too. C is negligent. D and F are extreme for now and G is valid but maybe see if you can resolve this situation locally first.

22 CDF

C shows initiative for your practice and ensures safety for your patients too. D ensures that you are working in accordance with your professional duty of care by raising the concern with your team members. F ensures the healthcare professional's senior is aware of the situation too, to advise and aid any further action required. A is unethical. B is extreme at this stage. E does not allow you to carry out root canals that will affect your clinical development this year. G is very similar to F; however, F is better as you gain advice and help. H is correct but does not tackle the unethical approach of what your educational supervisor and principal dentist is doing.

23 AEH

You have a professional duty of care to all patients and to the GDC to ensure that all members of your team are appropriately qualified and have the mandatory continuing professional development hours. Highlighting the issue to the principal is vital – he is in charge of all aspects of the practice and it is his duty to rectify anything that the GDC may deem as negligent, so A and E are correct. Highlighting and using this scenario to learn and reflect as a team will encourage all members to be compliant with GDC standards, especially keeping CPD up to date. B and G are extreme for now; C is negligent. F is unnecessary at this stage. D is valid; however, it does not show any initiative or action.

24 AEF

When considered together, A, E and F are the best combination, although B is valid. If you are telling the practice principal, at least the main provider for the practice is aware and can act accordingly. The GDC and CQC need to be reported to if the nurse does not register, so for now C and H can be dismissed. G is unethical and D is unnecessary as the wider practice does not need to be involved at this stage – especially if the practice principal has been notified.

25 ACD

Reassurance and communication are vital. This might be seen as confidentiality breach by the patient, so A needs to be done immediately. Follow-up appointments with this patient may be necessary if a complaint occurs. In B, by alerting many members of the team, you are causing a stir; for now this could be handled between you and the patient. C is useful for further learning and development; other senior members of the team can contribute their own experiences here and, as a team, you can reflect on this scenario. D is valid as a foundation dentist as ePDP will allow for written reflection and you can use this as a clinical audit topic – for example, medical history, confidentiality. E is valid; however, it is not as important as A. F and H are improper, rude and unnecessary. G could be valid in the future but usually only if a complaint arises.

26 BCD

B is good. It would be necessary to leave the room to call your educational supervisor, to calm down and to seek advice as soon as possible as this is quite an extreme event. D ensures that the patient is correctly handled and reassured and all dento-legal aspects are covered; B may need to occur to ensure full and contemporaneous advice is given on the day. All other options are valid and correct; however, B, C and D together are the best options covering all aspects of this scenario.

A – has not handled reassuring the patient or dento-legal options, nor has it involved the wider team;

E – has not dealt with dento-legal options or involved wider team and also suggests to the patient that all she can do is complain;

F – has not dealt with dento-legal options;

G – has not reassured the patient, has not dealt with the scenario at hand, and did not involve calling in your educational supervisor or wider team members;

H – has not told the patient or explained what has occurred; it has not reassured her or dealt with dento-legal issues.

27 BCF

B is a very good option as this is the most practical, clinical approach to rectify your mistake. You can also write in your clinical contemporaneous notes that you tried to remove the file unsuccessfully. C is a second-best answer; radiographically, you can also explain to the patient, diagnose the extent of blockage or fracture of file and radiographs also make up the notes or they can be used to send in a referral to a specialist endodontist. F is obvious; however, it must be stated as the patient's best interest always comes first and you have a duty of care to communicate effectively with all patients. A, E and H are irrelevant and negligent. D is irrelevant as you need to handle the situation now, not next week. G is valid but not yet and not with regard to the other answers – B, C and F act best when considered together.

28 DEF

F allows the correct member of staff to deal with the nurse and receptionist in conjunction with any practice policies in place. E ensures that the wider team knows the importance of teamworking and D ensures that you have taken the initiative in finding a solution to this problem. These answers are best when considered together. It is not your responsibility to deal with team animosity so the other options are not valid.

29 AEF

This is a very difficult position to be in; however, you must act to help your replacement and ensure the best for your patients and team. By telling the student throughout in a polite manner, as A suggests, then at the end of being shadowed her feedback may not be so much of a shock. Giving specific examples, as E suggests, is good as the patient can then reflect and learn from these areas of concern and F also allows the student to discuss the feedback with you and your educational supervisor (her future educational supervisor). B is valid but waiting until the end and doing so privately may cause the student to feel you are being unfair, especially if she had no prewarning and there are no other members of the team to witness the conversation. C does not allow the student an opportunity for fair discussion or opportunity to reflect. D is also valid but F ensures that your educational supervisor is a part of the process. G is true; however, it is acting in the best interest of the new DFT and you would want her to have a comfortable year ahead. Other colleagues do not need to become involved as this is confidential feedback for the student to learn from.

30 CDE

Practice policy would require any issues to be reported to the named person in charge, as C suggests. You can also take any written logs of missing items or dates and days the chair does not work to this person, or the principal, as D states. It might be important for the wider team to be fully aware of the events that have led to you raising these concerns, as E suggests. Whinging and moaning do not show initiative nor does sending official complaints to the GDC.

31 ABC

Vulnerable adults are a safeguarding issue, no matter whom or who is abusing them – all members of the team should be trained in this. Stop the situation before any further damage occurs, as A states. The practice manager needs to be informed, predominantly for further training and to gain a full insight into the scenario. D–H are not applicable in this scenario, so the best other option is C to ensure that all other team members are not also acting in such a manner. This would lead to further learning, reflection or an audit to reach gold standards of care.

32 CEF

Your obligation is to the GDC, so if you witness any malpractice or a scenario escalates higher than local level, as a professional you must raise any concerns. Signing shows complete disregard for this rule so A and D can be disregarded. Not signing but continuing to work without expressing your view, as B suggests, is deemed unprofessional. C, E and F are best when considered together, although H and G are valid statements.

33 AED

A is correct as all deaneries ensure a minimum of study days per year to graduate. E should have been done earlier, so in this instance ensure future dates are blocked off too. D is vital as it can help with advice on what to do next. B is unethical. C does not solve your problem as you will be short a study day. F is irrelevant and does not solve any problem. G is not applicable as this is an administrative organizational issue and H is untrue as no one is breaking the law.

34 BEF

The patient comes first. As B suggests, attend to the patient, make notes and, if you can, take photos – this will aid your notekeeping at the time and date of the examination. E is imperative, especially as a foundation dentist, because your educational supervisor and wider team can aid in helping you through this case. F shows good professionalism and a whole patient-care approach. A, G and H are halfhearted options and do not fully deal with the issue at hand. C would be applicable if the patient was a child. D is unprofessional and ignores the issue of the patient's consent.

35 BCE

To deal with the scenario, you need a trained member of staff to assist, as B states. E will be done after the patient is stabilized, which will be necessary in terms of taking this further as C states. B, C and E are best when considered together. A does not deal with the nurse's further training. D is not putting the patient's best interest first. F is unprofessional. G is extreme and H is not a standard means of delivering postoperative care with glucose water.

36 BDG

A dental practice has to act as a team so no member should be stressed or victimized. B is a good option as senior administrative staff can aid you. D allows the junior receptionist to present her case appropriately without just speculating and G shows a proactive approach in solving this issue. A staff meeting, as A suggests, could lead to further issues – ganging up or even conflict. C is unnecessary for a small staffing issue. E involves making an accusation without having evidence of your findings. F is not acting in the best interest of the team. H is valid but in this scenario, B, D and G are best considered together.

37 CDH

Criticism from your nurse should be accepted, so ensure you take her feedback seriously. D shows that you have reflected on her input; C then allows for further development and H will aid you in being taught how you can improve clinically. You should not ignore her as A states. B is similar. E is wrong as the nurse is helping you develop as a practitioner. F is not a fair representation of your work – three patients cannot judge your clinical ability. G is valid; however, it is probably more beneficial to speak to your TPD, who can aid you with your professional development.

38 DEG

By advising another practitioner you are acting in the best interests of the team and looking out for their professionalism so you should opt for D as one of the answers. B is also a good answer but D is better. C is valid but not at the moment as you need to give the associate a chance to come clean. F and H are unprofessional. E and G are the best options in this scenario – indemnity providers will give you the following steps to take and speaking to the associate on his arrival involving the wider team will hopefully ensure this never occurs again.

39 ABF

Explain and apologize; refer to secondary care and make contemporaneous notes on the entire scenario, as A, B and F state. C is not applicable – an opinion is needed from a specialist in secondary care. D is negligent. E is unnecessary as this is not an incident and just needs good clinical notes. G and H both may be valid but in this case it is assumed that a specialist in secondary care will prescribe accordingly.

40 ABE

Firstly, sympathize with your patient and assure him that you will endeavour to help him as B states. As A states, involve your educational supervisor as soon as possible and carry out all necessary investigations before referring to secondary care for an opinion. Always review patients like these in two weeks as E states. You should be able to handle a situation like this without intervention from your indemnity provider. D is valid too, but it is not the highest priority as A, B and E are. F is valid but E is better and G and H are very relaxed answers.

41 BDE

Medical emergencies are a mandatory CPD requirement to be addressed by all those registered with the GDC, so bring this up as soon as possible as B suggests. If you audit the CPD of the practice, this will allow you to use this as a means of proof to bring up at a practice meeting as D states. E is proactive and will help resolve this matter further giving the associate the tools to better himself for the future. A is negligent. C is a good statement but D is more appropriate as an audit gives specific examples and timings and forms a written log. F is extreme. G is inappropriate at the moment.

42 ACE

Any complaint may need indemnity input and your educational supervisor should be made aware about the complaint as A states. B is good but A is a better option as it includes your educational supervisor. C is the best option as it takes a proactive approach and allows you to empathize with the patient whose expectations were not being met. E needs to be done from a dento-legal viewpoint and ensuring that you experience further development in learning from an audit. D and H imply an easy way out without actually dealing with the patient's concerns. F may be how you feel; however it is unprofessional and no complaint should be dismissed. G should be included in your future plan; however A, C and E are the best options in this scenario.

43 BCF

You need a staff member who can assist you, so B needs to be done as soon as possible. Future learning is imperative, especially for the nurse who was unsure of what to do, so C is a good option. This leaves F, which is how to deal with the scenario and the patient whose needs should be acted upon in his best interest. You need to follow the resuscitation guidelines and calling 999 is not first on the list yet, so A can be ruled out. It is not your responsibility to train the nurse in basic life support, so D is not applicable. E is valid but BCF is more important. G is negligent. H is extreme.

44 CDF

You need to call your indemnity provider, speak to your educational supervisor and write good clinical notes, especially from a dento-legal perspective – these three options are best when considered together as CDF. A, E, G and H are negligent. B is good but your TPD is not in practice with you day in and out. He should not be making decisions for you; you are still a dental practitioner and should be in charge of your patients' diagnosis.

45 ABF

Always prepare yourself to treat patients using all your knowledge so you can act in their best interest. It is dangerous and unprofessional to treat patients with a complicated medical history about which you are not knowledgeable. A and F are therefore imperative. In the future you need to be prepared so B is a great option for further development. C and G is unethical and negligent. D is not applicable – you need to ensure you treat patients in their best interest and writing down your negligence does not justify you being negligent in the first place. E is a very good option but F is better as you can revise materials on your own in depth. You should not be using an old BNF as in H – all professional development should be kept up to date with the most up-to-date sources.

46 ABD

Deal with this scenario locally first, so speaking to the practice manager, as A states, is a good option. B is the next best option as your TPD will be trained to aid you further in this situation. D is actually a very respectable answer; if you have the confidence then approaching your educational supervisor directly would be beneficial. Understandably, this is a scenario that needs to be handled with tact so involvement of others is justified. C is extreme for now as there could be a solution to your concerns. Do not become introverted as E and G suggest. Do not justify your educational supervisor's actions as F suggests. Do not avoid the situation, as this is your year to learn – so do not do as H states.

47 ABC

You have every right to speak to social services as physical violence has been witnessed. You should also write a full record of this incident and of any staff members witnessing the event – so A and B are vital. In terms of handling the situation, include the wider team, which would include your educational supervisor, practice manager and any reception staff, to coordinate what you all do next, as C suggests. D, G and H are negligent and you should not be ignoring such a scenario, especially if a patient's safety is at risk. E is valid but, at present, a whole-team approach needs to be taken. F is also valid; however, in this situation you are justified in calling social services directly and this seems more important and in the patient's best interest. After A, B and C have been done, your indemnity provider should be called for further guidance.

48 ADE

Protocol requires a chest X-ray, so A comes first. Calling your educational supervisor for assistance is necessary especially if you are not confident (as you should be) with local protocol for bur retrieval, so D is a very good option. Lastly, E is obvious but necessary especially from a dento-legal perspective. B is dangerous as you cannot control suction and this will block the patient's airways. The first half of C is good; however, you should not carry on with treatment; you should stabilize the patient and send the patient for a chest X-ray. F implies that you are not dealing with the patient's safety but are just dealing with the administrative side – it also involves taking no action to rectify this situation. G and H are negligent.

49 ADE

Patient safety is an issue here and a multidisciplinary approach must be taken, as D suggests. A is important so that you are regularly seeing the patient and can hopefully encourage other options for the patient including counselling services. With increased recall you can manage any head and neck areas that may have been lacerated by the patient and look for any signs of self-harm. It is in your remit to give cessation advice, as E states. This is a very proactive approach. F and G are unprofessional and unsympathetic. H could be seen as rude and obnoxious instead of caring. B is applicable – however, you must look at the case as a whole. There are a lot of issues here and the patient has admitted self-harming; hence the patient's safety is definitely at risk so, in this scenario, including the GP is justified. However, in other scenarios you may not be able to do so without patient consent. Consent can only be breached when the patient's safety is seriously at risk or the wellbeing of society is at risk.

50 ABC

A complaint has been made; therefore the standard complaint protocol must be maintained, which is A, B and C. D and G are unprofessional. E is applicable but not yet – a thorough investigation needs to occur first. F is valid in history taking but could be deemed as accusatory. H is very unprofessional and instead of caring for the patient it suggests that you are not taking the complaint seriously.

51 AEF

The GDC regulations state that an appropriate interpreter must be given to any patients who do not speak English. As a team, come up with a plan to implement this idea as E states. A's survey is similar to a patient questionnaire or audit to ensure that many patients need this action. F is a brilliant option as shows it initiative and would help those finding it difficult with language barriers. B, D and H are unethical. C is very extreme and neglects English-speaking patients. G is not applicable.

52 ABD

Practices have to be accessible to all patients. This is a legal issue and A is valid. Including the wider team is important and D should be implemented immediately. B will help you move forward with this scenario, especially if you are a foundation dentist and find it difficult to raise this concern. C is very extreme and you should not be expected to fund, organize and execute the ramp installation. E and G are unethical as you know a ramp is a legal requirement. F is unethical. H is disregarding the issue at hand.

53 ABE

Mistakes happen. Stay calm (not as H suggests) and apologize to the patient as A states. Ask your nurse to call your educational supervisor to advise further if you are finding it hard to communicate effectively with the patient, as B suggests. If you cannot complete any treatment on the side you have anaesthetized then book the patient in at a later date when you can treat the other side, as E states. C may not be a very applicable option, as the patient should not be having two ID blocks, leaving him numb and unable to eat or speak. D is valid and you would not be entirely wrong in choosing this option; however, when considered together A, B and E are better suited as D is quite similar to B. F is unprofessional and does not have much relevance to the scenario. G is also a good option to do throughout your DF1 year; however, again, it has no relevance to the scenario.

54 ABC

You need to follow the resuscitation guidelines here, which, coincidently enough, are A, B and C! D, E and H are negligent and basic life support is a mandatory verified CPD, which should be updated annually, so leaving the patient in this state would have very serious consequences in front of the GDC.

55 ACD

The most valid answer is A. This is a direct safety issue for a child and you must make the child-protection lead aware of this scenario with your notes, which will form the basis for any investigations needed, and a letter to the social services. B is a very good answer; however, A is better and includes the notetaking. C is an excellent option as your educational supervisor can guide you through the process and can also attend in the surgery as a second healthcare professional to witness this case. D is necessary to ensure you take the correct route in helping your patient. E is negligence. You need to take any emotion out of this scenario and just concentrate on what is best for your patient, so F and G are inappropriate. H is not valid.

56 BCE

Your TPD will help you with this scenario as it is putting your clinical experience at risk. Clinicians should be confident in oral surgery – so B is a good option. If you can confront your educational supervisor this would be very helpful, especially at a time where you can use the situation as an example, as C states. E is a whole-team approach and might help the educational supervisor begin to help himself; it also ensures that the team will check up on him regularly. A and D are not necessary yet – it is best to deal with the issue privately first before embarrassing the educational supervisor in front of all the other staff members. The GDC does not need to be involved until local measures have been taken, so F can be eliminated first. G does not help your clinical ability as you may need your educational supervisor for support. H is negligent and not helping the entire team.

57 BDE

B, D and E cover all aspects of complaint handling – good notes and a whole-team approach. The practice manager should deal with the complaint with you. Audit complaints and include educational supervisors for future support. A is unethical; you need to ensure that the practice knows about the complaints. Writing a complaint alone, as a foundation dentist, is not advisable, so C is not a viable option. F may be applicable in the future, if a breakdown of trust has occurred; however, you cannot pass the buck – you must ensure that you are able to handle complaints logically and with a good outlook for your relationship with your patients. G and H are unprofessional and go against the GDC guidelines.

58 BCD

All new materials need to have formal training in use, so B and C are necessary. You must consider risk and benefit and which resin may be applicable to each individual, so D is an excellent answer here. You are not limiting yourself to one individual resin material. A suggests that all you will be using is the resin composite and nothing else and E suggests you will not even trial the product at all, even though it may be a fantastic new material to use. Your flatmate's discussion, in F, is not a valid option. Calling the GDC is not applicable in this scenario. G is irrelevant.

59 BCD

Your colleague needs more advice from occupational health, as B states. C is very useful because indemnity providers will suggest the best route of action to take. The colleague can speak to his educational supervisor, as D states; however, this may or may not be compulsory and an indemnity provider could provide further advice on this. With regard to A, the GDC does not need to know yet. You should not advise the colleague on any dento-legal aspects as E, F and G suggest. H is not necessary – it is better your colleague speaks to his own indemnity provider.

60 ADG

You need to reassure patients without commenting on another practitioner's conduct without a full investigation or advice from other bodies – A ensures that the patient is at ease and a further conversation will occur. G ensures that, with dento-legal considerations in mind, the patient's conversation is written down – this could escalate into a complaint. Finally, as D states, you allow the patient time to think about matters with the principal in attendance. Do not comment on the principal's conduct as B and F state, or ask your nurse to, as C states. E is unprofessional and not sympathetic to the patient. H is irrelevant to the scenario – however you should not be telling patients a root canal will be a 100% success.

61 ACD

You cannot work alone, so either a locum should be arranged, as A states, or patients should be cancelled, which in an ideal situation you do not want to occur (B). So, prioritize patients who need to be seen and those who are new patients or routine exams, as C suggests. Your educational supervisor can be called and notified about the situation, as D states, especially if it leaves you in a difficult position. E and H are unprofessional and not working in the best interest of the patients booked – however if all options fail then, yes, the practice should be closed and patients cancelled. The CQC do not need to be called in regards to this (F) – try to deal with issues locally first. Future reflection is necessary as G states; however A, C and D are the best options for now when considered together.

62 CDE

C is a good diplomatic answer. D shows initiative and the indemnity provider can advise on the route to take in handling this scenario. E ensures that the treating dentist now handles this grievance further. A is valid; however, you should at least listen or empathize with the patient. You should not comment on the grievance until investigations have taken place so you can eliminate B. The patient is not to blame and it is unprofessional to suggest this to the patient at all as F and G state. H is negligent and unethical.

63 CFH

You cannot treat patients or plan treatment fully without a medical history – so H and C are suggested. If you cannot relay this information due to the patient's attitude you need to implement F, as senior colleagues are experienced in handling more difficult patients. With regard to A, you cannot dismiss patients. B suggests that treatment can be done, which is not true as a full medical history is needed for *any* treatment to take place. D is irrelevant. E is unethical. G is unprofessional as you are just passing the patient on and not dealing with the issue at hand.

64 EGH

This is clinical negligence. This question is particularly difficult and there is not much wrong with the statements in a lot of the answers so you must think about what is best when they are considered together. Write your notes up properly, with all clinical findings and any radiograph reports (E), tell the patient your findings and explain why you will not be fitting the crown (G) and then take the matter forward with the associate (H), including the wider team. A is negligence. B is a good option; however, G is a better option than B alone. C suggests that you are not going to bring up the fact there is caries and allow the patient to have the crown fitted without being told. Calling your educational supervisor in is an option; however, if you can diagnose caries clinically, then you can explain your findings to both your educational supervisor and associate together. The practice does not need to be told about this issue yet – only if staff need more training can this scenario be brought up as the associate may rectify the mistake and treatment plan for his patient better

65 ABD

Try to solve the matter locally first, as A suggests. If you cannot, then proceed to speak to your TPD, as B states, and then include the wider team, as D suggests. However, H is inappropriate as you need to be the one speaking to your educational supervisor about how you feel. With regard to C, this is not a GDC matter. Do not fall behind, as E suggests; try to rectify the issue and move forward to gain the best out of your year. This is not the other FD's fault so do not embarrass him or yourself by complaining about his progress as F states. Your undergraduate tutors cannot implement any changes within the FD year; however, they are always available to help and talk if necessary (G).

66 BEA

This error is not of your own making but you will need to lead on how it is managed. You need to speak with your educational supervisors to explain what has happened. It is important that you try to work with the rest of the team in correcting this diary mistake so that your patients are looked after and not cancelled. It is also important that you inform your TPD about what has occurred so that all parties are aware and have enough notice to resolve the situation. Be aware that option H is unprofessional.

67 ABC

The importance of time management cannot be overstated. Don't try to be a hero and see all these patients yourself. You will overrun, keep patients waiting and prevent staff from leaving on time. Forewarning your educational supervisor of the situation, so she is aware of the need to be around if help is needed, is a much better way of managing the situation. It demonstrates good leadership skills and consideration for the team. By asking your educational supervisor and other dentists in the practice if they are able to fit in a few of the older children, the whole team will finish on time. There should be a discussion at the next practice meeting to prevent this happening again.

68 ACD

Conflict among colleagues, especially in front of patients, is unprofessional and could give the practice a poor reputation and erode goodwill. Ask the practice manager to speak to both parties seeking a resolution and do not become directly involved in the issues. Speak to the principal, asking her to bring up the importance of working as a team and respecting one another at the next practice meeting. This will have a more positive effect on everyone and enable the practice to be seen as a professional enterprise by patients.

69 ADE

It is your duty to safeguard all your patients. If you have tried to explain reasonable options to the parents who then go onto choose options that are not in the interests of the child then you may wish to suggest a second opinion. Speak to your educational supervisor privately with regard to this case, asking for detailed advice and ask if he could see the parents to offer a second opinion. Ensure that you note all conversations down in contemporaneous note form. Always ensure that you explain all outcomes and options to the parents, giving your professional opinion on the matter.

70 ACH

It is not your fault that the patient has developed a cold sore. It is, however, important that you acknowledge the inconvenience caused to the patient by the fact that you are unable to see him today. You need to explain that this decision is out of your hands as it is practice policy not to treat patients with cold sores. Explain this is routine in the dental setting due to the contagious nature of the Herpes Simplex Virus (HSV) virus. Advise the patient to purchase over-the-counter topical acyclovir and analgesics if necessary. Rebook the patient in next week, when the cold sore should have healed.

71 CEF

Patients who are under the influence of drugs are unable to give consent. Asking for help from your educational supervisor will ensure that a second opinion is given to the patient and you will all be able to work together to ensure the safety of the patient. Do not be afraid to ask the patient directly for an up-to-date medical history ensuring to ask if he uses recreational drugs. This demonstrates that you have the patient's best interests at heart and that you are ensuring safety for the patient. Make sure that you record all conversations down in contemporaneous notes.

72 ABC

Part of your job as a team leader and professional is to ensure the safety of your team. All team members have a right to work in a safe and nonthreatening environment. Asking your patient to wait in your surgery whilst you help the reception deal with this patient is the most appropriate action. If possible, try to move the patient to a side room to discuss matters further away from other patients. If you are unable to diffuse the situation, call for help from the principal and always be ready to call the police if violence is involved.

73 ADF

Any employer will be annoyed if an employee is consistently late. If patients constantly have to be rescheduled, they will soon get fed up and may go to another practice. There is no point in becoming upset – you need to resolve the issue, so explain your predicament to the educational supervisor and practice principal, trying to put a more appropriate plan in place. You should also speak to your TPD in regards to the whole scenario to help advise further. Don't take the comments so personally; the principal has a business to run and you have a responsibility to treat patients in a professional manner.

74 ABD

The conduct of the nurse is unprofessional and you should discuss this with her at the first opportunity. You should withdraw from the social group and discuss the matter with the principal as this will reflect badly on the practice. You should use the opportunity for discussion at the next practice meeting to outline the dangers of doing this on social media. The nurse may not realize what the potential problems are with social media issues so you will be helping her by outlining the pitfalls.

75 ACE

It is against the law to discriminate against disabled people and prosecution could result if the practice continues with this misguided philosophy. As difficult as it may be, you should call CQC and ask them to intervene as proper facilities for disabled people should be made available. Speak to your TPD and your educational supervisor for advice.

CHAPTER 8

How to write a dental CV

Introduction

Your CV is a document that enables potential employers to learn basic facts about you and your job-related experiences, achievements and education. It is a reflection of you. Writing a CV is a skill and as such it requires planning and discipline. There are many web sites that offer help and support but ultimately your CV should be succinct, informative and aimed directly at the job for which you are applying.

Most dental undergraduates who have entered university straight from school often feel that they have very little to write about in terms of their acquired skills and employment history. This is untrue! I have spent many years looking through undergraduate CVs and the first thing I look at is hobbies and interests. The next thing I look at is *any* employment history – especially voluntary. This yields a wealth of information upon which an undergraduate CV can be based.

At any stage of a career, I would advise that two CVs are kept. One should be a *'chronological CV'* that documents everything that relates to work that you have done (dental or otherwise). The other is the CV for the job for which you are applying. The first will enable you to draw upon relevant experiences for the second.

The Dental Foundation Interview Guide: with Situational Judgement Tests, First Edition.
Zahid Siddique, Shivana Anand and Helena Lewis-Greene.
© 2017 John Wiley & Sons, Ltd. Published 2017 by John Wiley & Sons, Ltd.

Although a CV is seldom required for the DF1 process, some 'meet-and-greet' teams ask that you bring your CV to the meeting. What is the DF1 educational supervisor looking for? The answer is the valued dental competencies upon which the DF1 process is based. Look at the record sheets for clinical communication and professionalism and leadership scenarios and you will see the following listed:

1 Empathy and sensitivity.
2 Reassurance and problem solving.
3 Information sharing.
4 Generic clinical communication.
5 Appropriate professional attitudes.
6 Clinical knowledge and expertise.
7 Presentation of clinical options (communication).
8 Understanding of evidence-informed practice.

Often, when I check a CV, I read through lists of skills. *'I am well disciplined, focused, empathetic and a good team member.'* This tells the reader nothing about you as an individual. Why would they employ you? If you tell the reader how you obtained your skills, you personalize your experiences and capture the reader's imagination.

Format

An excellent format for a dental undergraduate CV should include the following sections:

- **Personal statement** – ensure that you draw upon your experiences, both personally and as a student, to highlight your skills. A personal statement should succinctly reveal to the reader your strengths and weaknesses. What have you gained over the 5 years as a student? How has your clinical experience helped you communicate with patients and colleagues? What experiences have enabled you to become a better team member and what skills have helped you understand equality and diversity? Creating a personal statement is not an easy task and takes time. You need to reflect and really understand yourself as a person. It takes courage to admit weaknesses but no one expects you to know it all. Your aim is to be a safe beginner.
- **Key skills – don't just list them!** Work out what enabled you to achieve them. If you have had limited work experience then draw upon your leisure activities and hobbies. Classic examples include dance, music and sport. If you have engaged in any of these activities you will have needed to be **well disciplined**, **well organized** and **resilient.** You will have learned from an early age how to work together with others to maximize performance as a **team**. Any cultural experiences will have helped your **communication and interpersonal skills** as well as understand the meaning of **equality and diversity**. If you come from a background where your family has been self-employed, has this **motivated** you to follow in their footsteps? Did you help your family with their business? Did this involve you and **interacting and communicating with the public?**

- **Strengths** – once these skills have been identified you can use them to highlight how they will help you in your job. For example:

  My extracurricular activities imposed time restraints upon me and I have had to learn to organize my work time well.

  I found that I had to really listen to people in my retail job. This enabled me to understand what they really wanted

  Having mentored younger students / young people within my community, I have developed good listening and empathy skills'

- **Weaknesses** – do **not** be afraid to discuss your weaknesses and limitations. Make it clear that you often had to seek help from tutors or bosses when situations became tough. This highlights **responsibility**, especially where patients are concerned. **Knowing your limitations** in dentistry is hugely important as it protects everyone. Admit that there are aspects of dentistry that are demanding and challenging. You aim to use your DF1 year to learn how to improve your work and increase your confidence.

- **Work experience** –any work experience will be valuable to you for your CV and future career. Work experience enables you to understand organization, teamwork, discipline, responsibility, professionalism, empathy and communication. Your work experience may also have helped you understand how not to do things. We usually learn more from mistakes! One of the most valuable work experiences is in a dental practice. Very often when I ask students about their jobs they say, 'well I only work in a dental practice.' What could be more valuable for future careers than to witness and experience it first hand? Very often students ask if they should list their undergraduate clinical experiences. I think that this is important but it must be done in a concise and general way as it can eat into valuable CV space.

- **Voluntary and nondental work experience** – voluntary work has become increasingly important within recruitment as it shows willingness help build stronger communities and sends a clear message that there are more important things to you than just making money. It can provide key contacts via networking and shows commitment to caring for people. It can also provide key skills, which can be useful later on and can also bridge gaps in CVs. Many employers are themselves contributors to charities and this would show them your humanitarian side. Voluntary work is also important as it reveals something of your character and personality. A recent student wrote:

  The school was for children of a wide range of learning difficulties / special needs and my role was to help the children in class with both learning and recreational activities from literacy skills to creative skills in the form of art and design and music. This increased my interpersonal skills and gave me an insight into how to communicate effectively with children and people with special needs.

This wonderful experience also highlighted the caring, empathetic and sensitive side of the student, which he could draw upon in his professional capacity as a dentist:

- **Memberships** – this will confirm your indemnity and commitment to professional associations.
- **Languages** – these are hugely important at a time where many people of all races live closely together and communication has become a key GDC domain.
- **Hobbies and interests** – again this reveals much about personality and character. It also acts as a barometer of the life / work balance. Dentistry is a highly pressurized profession and being able to have a good work / life balance will reveal much about your maturity.

Some dos and don'ts

1 Remember that no one CV fits all. You should tailor your CV for the job.
2 Read the job specification and highlight the key skills. Do you have them? How did you get them?
3 Make sure that your CV is neat and clear enough for a recruiter to scan and understand it quickly.
4 Make sure that your personal details are current and that you have included a current address, landline and mobile telephone numbers.
5 Keep your personal statement short and to the point.
6 Keep the CV to two pages including references.
7 Choose a clear, professional font to ensure that your CV can be read easily.
8 Avoid typing mistakes at all costs. A simple spell check is not enough; ask someone else to proofread your finished CV.

The meet and greet

✓ Dress smart.
✓ Be punctual.
✓ Do your research – visit the practice web site, familiarize yourself with location, specialists available, distance in miles, DF1 number and educational supervisors.
✓ Get together a CV – some meet and greets have an interview for 20 minutes where both trainees and educational supervisors get to rank their preferences; others have an informal chat.

Some useful questions to ask

✓ Parking availability.
✓ Working hours.
✓ Number of surgeries.

✓ Number of clinical staff.

✓ Rotating or set nurse.

✓ Hygiene / therapist – can you refer to them for treatment?

✓ Endodontics: hand files or rotary availability.

✓ Number of patients seen per average day.

✓ Type of patients? High needs? Ask current FDs what their clinical experience has been like.

✓ Specialists / special interests.

✓ What do they do as a practice socially?

✓ Clinical audit time.

✓ What are they looking for in a trainee?

✓ Ask the FDs what their plan is after DF1. This gives you an indication if the practice helps with DF2 applications or associate jobs.

✓ Commute: easy to get to? Local schools in the area?

✓ Types of tutorials run in the practice, how are they delivered.

✓ What do they expect from you – clinical quota wise?

Index

The Dental Foundation Interview Guide: with Situational Judgement Tests, First Edition.
Zahid Siddique, Shivana Anand and Helena Lewis-Greene.
© 2017 John Wiley & Sons, Ltd. Published 2017 by John Wiley & Sons, Ltd.